A Practical Guide to
Real-Time
Office Sonography
in Obstetrics
and Gynecology

A Practical Guide to Real-Time Office Sonography in Obstetrics and Gynecology

Robert V. Giglia, R.T., R.D.M.S.
Kara L. Mayden, R.T., R.D.M.S.
and
Norbert Gleicher, M.D.
Rush Medical College and
Mount Sinai Hospital and Medical Center of Chicago
Chicago, Illinois

With the collaboration of
Haim Elrad, M.D., and Jan Friberg, M.D., Ph.D.

PLENUM MEDICAL BOOK COMPANY
New York and London

Library of Congress Cataloging in Publication Data

Giglia, Robert V.
  A practical guide to real-time office sonography in obstetrics and gynecology.

  Includes bibliographies and index.
  1. Ultrasonics in obstetrics. 2. Generative organs, Female — Diseases — Diagnosis. 3. Diagnosis, Ultrasonic. I. Mayden, Kara L. II. Gleicher, Norbert. III. Title. [DNLM: 1. Genital Diseases, Female — diagnosis. 2. Pregnancy Complications — diagnosis. 3. Prenatal Diagnosis — methods. 4. Ultrasonic Diagnosis. WQ 209 G459p]
RG527.5.U48G54 1986   618   85-12033
ISBN-13: 978-0-306-41865-5   e-ISBN-13: 978-1-4615-8348-6
DOI: 10.1007/978-1-4615-8348-6

© 1986 Plenum Publishing Corporation
Softcover reprint of the hardcover 1st edition 1986
233 Spring Street, New York, N.Y. 10013

Plenum Medical Book Company is an imprint of Plenum Publishing Corporation

This book is dedicated to my parents, whose support and love made this book and my career possible.

Robert V. Giglia

I dedicate this book to my father and mother, who have inspired, guided, and encouraged me in my personal and professional evolution.

Kara L. Mayden

To my family.

Norbert Gleicher

Contents

PART II. REAL-TIME SONOGRAPHY IN GYNECOLOGY

Introduction

Real-time ultrasonography has entered office practice in obstetrics and gynecology. With increasing numbers of sonography systems entering the ambulatory office setting, obstetric sonography at a routine level (level I) has largely been the targeted area. Recent developments in gynecologic real-time sonography have, however, significantly enlarged the sphere of applicability of sonographic equipment in an office setting. The very rapid growth of follicular sonography in infertility assessment and management has made real-time sonography of increasing importance to the gynecologic practitioner. In office settings like the authors', gynecologic office sonography represents close to 50% of all ordered sonography.

This handbook of office sonography in obstetrics and gynecology was conceived to reflect these changes in practice patterns. This volume is not meant to replace standard sonography texts for the full-time sonographer but is instead directed toward the practicing obstetrician/gynecologist who uses real-time sonography in the office setting within the framework of daily practice. Technical comments were therefore restricted to a minimum, with practical advice and photographic examples taking their place.

Most of the sonographic real-time images were retrieved from the authors' own files. However, some were obtained through the generosity of friends and colleagues, for which we would like to extend acknowledgment and appreciation. Similar appreciation is extended to Dr. Haim Elrad and Dr. Jan Friberg, who also participated in the editorial process; to Sheila Martin, who performed superbly as our editorial assistant, a most difficult responsibility; and to Hilary Evans, our editor at Plenum Publishing Corporation.

Robert V. Giglia
Kara L. Mayden
Norbert Gleicher

Introduction

A Practical Guide to
Real-Time
Office Sonography
in Obstetrics
and Gynecology

Chapter 1
Indications for
Sonography

Indications for sonography have been only poorly defined in the literature. With increasing availability of ultrasound units, the use of sonography in obstetrics and gynecology has significantly increased. As occurs so frequently in medicine, such an increase in use at times leads to overuse and abuse of diagnostic modalities.

1.1. OBSTETRICS

A recent Consensus Development Conference, organized by the National Institutes of Health, strongly reaffirmed the fact that obstetric sonography should not be performed on a routine basis. While such a routine approach has its proponents, particularly in Europe, a more selective approach seems to make sense. Obstetric sonography should therefore only be performed if a specific indication exists.

1.2. GYNECOLOGY

No such recommendation for the application of sonography to gynecologic practice has been recently proposed. Recommendations referring to gynecology have been made by the American College of Obstetricians and Gynecologists (see Chapter 2) but are clearly outdated. The utilization of sonography in gynecologic practice has revolutionized the field. Nevertheless, it must always be remembered that sonography should under no circumstances replace either pelvic examination or histopathology. Sonography in gynecologic practice thus serves as an adjunct to older diagnostic means, not as a replacement.

Chapter 2
ACOG/AIUM Recommendations

2.1. AMERICAN COLLEGE OF OBSTETRICIANS AND GYNECOLOGISTS[1]

2.1.1. Primary Indications for the Use of Ultrasound in Obstetrics

1. Gestational age
2. Abnormalities of early pregnancy
3. Pre- and postamniocentesis studies
4. Fetal growth studies
5. Vaginal bleeding
6. Presentation of fetus
7. Multiple pregnancies
8. Congenital malformation
9. Determination of fetal lie (presentation)
10. Pelvic masses
11. Hydatidiform mole

2.1.2. Clinical Indications in Gynecology

1. Simple ovarian cysts
2. Tubo-ovarian abscesses
3. Extrauterine pregnancy
4. Dermoid cyst
5. Ascites
6. Location intrauterine device
7. Myomas
8. Ovarian tumors

2.2. AMERICAN INSTITUTE OF ULTRASOUND IN MEDICINE—SECTION OF OBSTETRICS AND GYNECOLOGY[2]

Diagnostic ultrasound has several applications in obstetrics and gynecology:

1. To determine fetal viability when abortion or intrauterine demise is suspected
2. To determine gestational age when there is a consistent discrepancy between clinical findings and the patient's dates
3. To locate the placenta when there is vaginal bleeding or when fetus is in an unstable lie

4. To evaluate a gestation at any stage when there is a discrepancy between uterine size and dates
5. Before amniocentesis
6. To monitor fetal growth when intrauterine growth retardation (IUGR) is suspected
7. When multiple gestation is suspected
8. When congenital anomalies are suspected
9. To determine fetal size in breech presentation
10. To evaluate amniotic fluid quantity
11. To evaluate post-term pregnancy
12. To evaluate possible molar pregnancies
13. As an adjunct to special procedures such as intrauterine transfusion, placental aspiration, and fetoscopy
14. To evaluate a pelvic mass during pregnancy

REFERENCES

1. *ACOG Tech Bull* 1981;63.
2. Paraphrased by Kremkau FW: How safe is obstetric ultrasound? *Contemporary OB/GYN* 1982;20:182.

Chapter 3
Principles of Real-Time
Sonography

3.1. PHYSICS

Real-time sonography is the branch of ultrasound that enables the investigator to observe dynamic, or moving, images during the scanning process.

3.1.1. Theory of Sound-Wave Propagation

Sound waves are directed into the body as a result of an electrical impulse that excites one or more piezoelectric crystal(s) within the transducer element. The crystal will expand and contract in response to this excitation; as a consequence, mechanical pressure waves are transmitted through the body. Sound waves travel within the tissues (1540 m/sec), and a portion are reflected back to the transducer when encountered by a boundary between two tissues (interface). The remaining sound waves continue through the tissue interface. The angle at which the sound waves strike the interface and the difference in density between the two tissues determine the amount of reflected sound. The best reflection of sound is achieved when the sound beam hits the target perpendicularly. The acoustic impedance (Z) is defined as the product of the propagation speed of sound (v) and the density of the tissues (p) ($Z = pv$). Two tissues with large differences in acoustic impedance can be easily differentiated from one another (e.g., bone versus amniotic fluid). Tissues with similar acoustic impedances may be difficult to easily distinguish with ultrasound (e.g., fetal liver versus kidney).[1-3]

3.1.2. Real-Time Equipment

The two most commonly used types of real-time equipment in obstetric and gynecologic ultrasound are linear and sector arrays.

Linear Array: This type of format will project a rectangular image. The piezoelectric crystals (64–128) are lined in sequence along the transducer head. The crystals are electronically pulsed and fired in predetermined sequences (4–5 crystals fired at a time). This constant emission of sound waves provides a moving, or cinematic, image.

Sector Array: The transmission of sound waves in the sector array is similar to that described for linear arrays. The transducer crystals, however, are arranged in a predetermined pie shape. The groups of crystals are fired in an arc pattern. Mechanical and phased arrays systems are commonly used.[4]

3.1.3. Common Applications of Real-Time Equipment

Linear Array: This format is commonly used in obstetric sonography. The large size of the transducer head allows for easy orientation and aids in obtaining fetal measurements.

Sector Array: Sector arrays are used both in obstetrics and in gynecology. The small size of the transducer head allows for placement of the transducer in the pelvis, thereby permitting assessment of pelvic anatomy.

REFERENCES

1. Kremkau FW: *Diagnostic Ultrasound: Physical Principles and Exercises,* New York, Grune & Stratton, 1980.
2. Ziskin MC: Basic physics of ultrasound, in Sanders RC, James AE Jr (eds): *Ultrasonography in Obstetrics and Gynecology,* East Norwalk, Conn, Appleton-Century-Crafts, 1977, pp 7–27.
3. Sanders RC: *Clinical Sonography: A Practical Guide.* Boston, Little, Brown, 1984, pp 3–18.
4. Blackwell R: New developments in equipment. *Clin Obstet Gynecol* 1983;10:3.

3.2. CLINICAL AND TECHNICAL CONSIDERATIONS

Clinical and technical considerations are difficult to summarize because of variations in equipment and patients. Some simple standards should, however, be followed. A thin patient or a child requires less penetration of the ultrasound beam. Consequently, a higher-frequency (3.5–5 MHz) transducer, which will increase the resolution, should be used when penetration is not a concern. Conversely, in the obese or third-trimester pregnant patient, in whom penetration of the ultrasound beam can be a problem, sacrificing some resolution for better penetration may be warranted. This can be accomplished by decreasing the frequency (3.0–2.25 MHz). A simple formula for these applications is presented in the following two alternatives:

A: ↑ frequency ↓ penetration ↑ resolution
B: ↓ frequency ↑ penetration ↓ resolution

The sonographic demonstration of structures, whether normal or abnormal, has specific characteristics. The sonographer should perform gain studies to determine these characteristics (see Fig. 3.2.1).

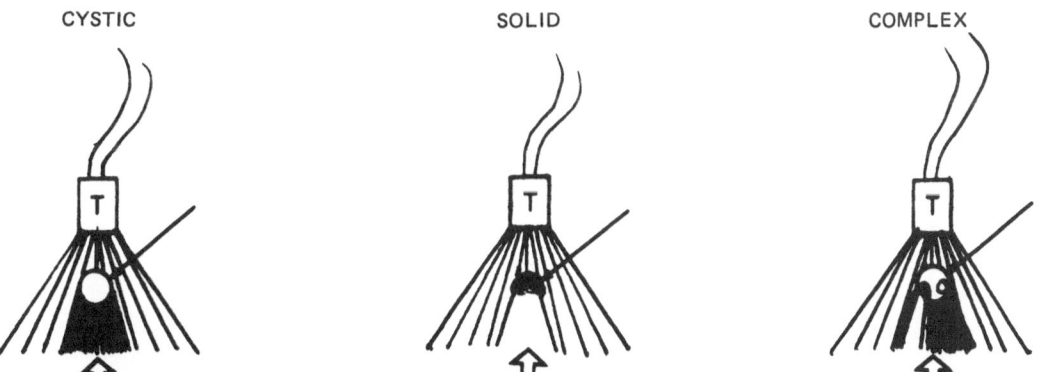

CYSTIC   SOLID   COMPLEX

FIG. 3.2.1. SONOGRAPHIC APPEARANCE OF STRUCTURES

Characteristics of cystic, solid, and complex structures as seen by sonography. Arrowhead points to transonicity or beam transmission, while arrow points to structure in question. (See also Section 21.2.) (Illustration by R. V. Giglia.)

If the appearance of the structure in question is compared with a known sonographic appearance, i.e., cyst versus urinary bladder, the acoustic characteristics are easily evaluated.

Once a mass or abnormal appearance has been visualized, an easy method of description is to use the formula SALT, which stands for

Size and shape
Acoustic characteristics (internal echo pattern)
Location (see Fig. 19.1.2)
Transonicity (posterior echo pattern)

Part I
Real-Time Sonography in Obstetrics

Chapter 4
Normal Fetal Anatomy

4.1. PRINCIPLES OF ROUTINE SCANNING

A recent National Institutes of Health (NIH) Consensus Development Conference evaluated the question of whether obstetric sonography should be routinely applied in every pregnancy. The consensus was that sonography should be restricted to those pregnancies in which a clear medical indication for the procedure exists. This handbook follows the NIH recommendations.

Obstetric sonography can be reported in various ways. A sample of a reporting sheet is presented in Fig. 4.1.1.

OBSTETRIC SONOGRAPHY REPORT

TO BE FILLED OUT BY REFERRING PHYSICIAN

PATIENT'S NAME: ____________
ADDRESS: ____________
____________ Zip ____________
TELEPHONE (Home): ____________
TELEPHONE (Business): ____________
DATE: ____________

Referring Physician: ____________
Address: ____________
____________ Zip ____________
Telephone: ____________
Patient before: No ______ Yes ______
Patient Billing: ______ Office Billing: ______

AGE: ______ PREGNANCY TEST: ______ (+) ______ (−) PARA: ______ LMP: ______

HX: By Dates: ____________ PREVIOUS SONO: Date: ______
By Size: ____________ BPD: ______
Placenta: ______
Amniotic Fluid: ______

When ordering the test, please indicate (x) which evaluation is to be performed.

______ LEVEL I (Routine OB) ______ LEVEL II (Target Imaging)

TO BE RECORDED BY PERINATAL TESTING CENTER

SONOGRAPHIC RESULTS

No. of Gestations ______ Fetal Heart Yes ____ No ____ Fetal Position ______

BPD= ______ CMS= ______ wks. Amniotic Fluid: ______

Femur Length= ______ CMS= ______ wks. Placental Location ______

Abd. Circ.= ______ CMS= ______ wks. Placental Grade ______

HEAD/ABD RATIO= ______

GESTATIONAL AGE ESTIMATED TO BE ______ to ______ WEEKS

COMMENTS: ____________

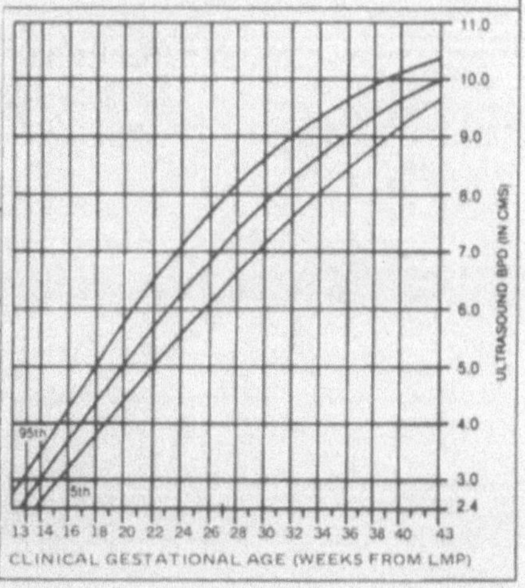

Thank you for referring this patient. Should you have any further questions, please do not hesitate to call us.

______ M.D.

FIG. 4.1.1. SAMPLE OBSTETRIC SONOGRAPHY REPORT

4.2. THE FETAL HEAD

4.2.1. Lateral Ventricles

- To find the lateral ventricles, one needs to identify the long axis of the fetus (spine or aorta). When the top of the fetal head comes into view, the transducer is rotated by 90°.

- The lateral ventricles appear as linear echoes equidistant from the central (falx) midline at a height just superior to the fetal biparietal diameter (BPD).

- Up to approximately 20–22 weeks, the lateral borders of the ventricles will usually fill more than half the lateral hemisphere and should therefore not be confused with early hydrocephaly. After 20–22 weeks, ventricles occupy proportionally less space and should be identifiable at no more than halfway between falx and lateral skull.

- Nomograms are available to measure the diameter of the ventricles. This is done by utilizing the following formula:

$$\frac{\text{Lateral ventricle (LV)}}{\text{Hemispheric width (HW)}} \times 100 = \text{LV/HW ratio}$$

See also Section 16.2.2 and Fig. 4.2.1.

4.2.2. Fetal Biparietal Diameter

- The level of the normal fetal biparietal diameter (BPD) is obtained inferiorly to the above-described level for the lateral ventricles (see Fig. 4.2.2). For further details concerning the BPD, see Section 7.2.

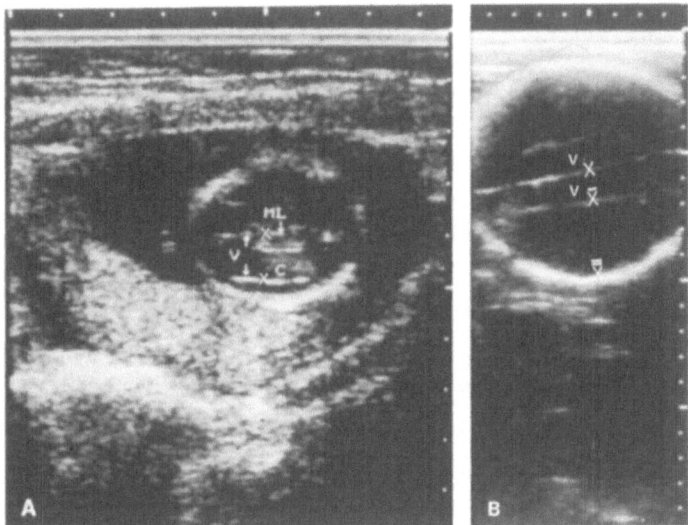

FIG. 4.2.1. NORMAL LATERAL VENTRICLES

(A) Transverse scan at the level of the lateral ventricles (V, arrows) in a 14–15-week gestation. Note the distance (calipers) of the ventricle from the midline (ML), which in early second trimester is considered within normal limits. Choroid plexus (C).

(B) Transverse scan through the fetal head at 34 weeks gestation, demonstrating the lateral ventricles (v). Note that the lateral border of the ventricle ($\bar{X}$) appears to be less than halfway between the midline (X) and the inner skull table ($\bar{\bar{X}}$). The lateral ventricular width (distance from X to $\bar{X}$) and the hemispheric width (X to $\bar{\bar{X}}$) can be determined and used to detect hydrocephalus.

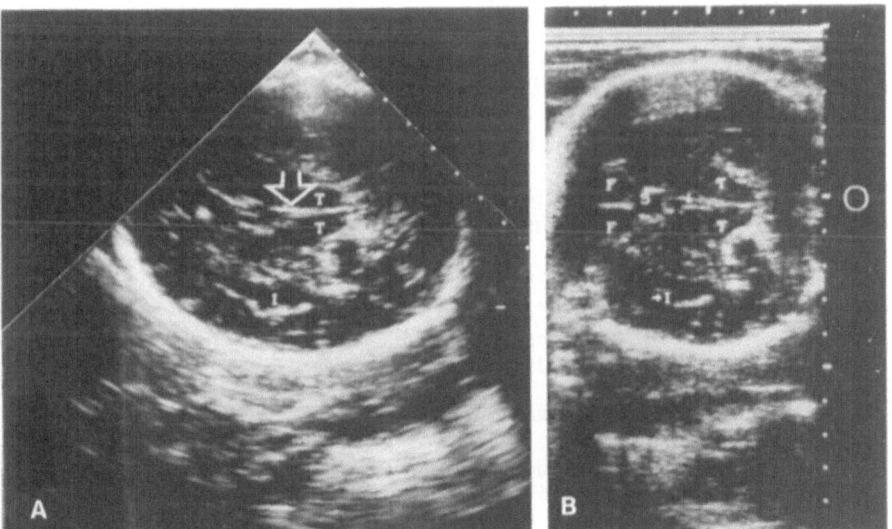

FIG. 4.2.2. THE FETAL HEAD AT THE HEIGHT OF THE BPD

(A) Transverse scan through the fetal cranium demonstrating the thalami (T), the midline (open arrow), and the sylvian fissure or insula (I). Pulsations visualized in the lateral cranial hemisphere will differentiate the sylvian fissure (I) from the lateral ventricle.

(B) Transverse scan depicting normal intracranial anatomy. Frontal horns of ventricles (F), occiput (O), septum pellucidum (S), third ventricle (arrow), thalami (T).

4.2.3. The Fetal Orbits

- The fetal orbits represent a landmark below the level of the fetal BPD.

- When the fetal position precludes measurement of the fetal BPD, fetal orbital measurements have been found useful for determination of fetal gestational age and the antenatal diagnosis of hypotelorism and hypertelorism.[1-3] (See also Section 7.2 and Fig. 4.2.3.)

REFERENCES

1. Jeanty P, Dramaix-Wilmet M, Van Gausbeke D, et al: Fetal ocular biometry by ultrasound. *Radiology* 1982;143:513.
2. Mayden KL, Tortora M, Berkowitz, RL, et al: Orbital diameters: A new parameter for prenatal diagnosis and dating. *Am J Obstet Gynecol* 1982;144:289.
3. Mayden KL: Orbital distance measurements: Techniques for prenatal diagnosis and dating. *Med Ultrasound* 1984;8:117.

4.2.4. The Fetal Face

- Resolution with modern real-time equipment has progressed to such an extent that detailed facial structures such as the ocular lens, the nasal septum, the maxilla, and the tongue can now be visualized (see Fig. 4.2.4).

- Consequently, it has been possible to diagnose antenatally facial abnormalities such as cleft lip and cleft palate.[4,5] (See Fig. 17.2.3.)

REFERENCES

4. Christ JE, Meninger MC: Ultrasonic diagnosis of cleft lip and cleft palate before birth. *Plast Reconstr Surg* 1981;6:854.
5. Chervenak FA, Tortora M, Mayden KL, et al: Median cleft face syndrome: Ultrasonic demonstration of cleft lip and hypertelorism. *Am J Obstet Gynecol* 1984;149:94.

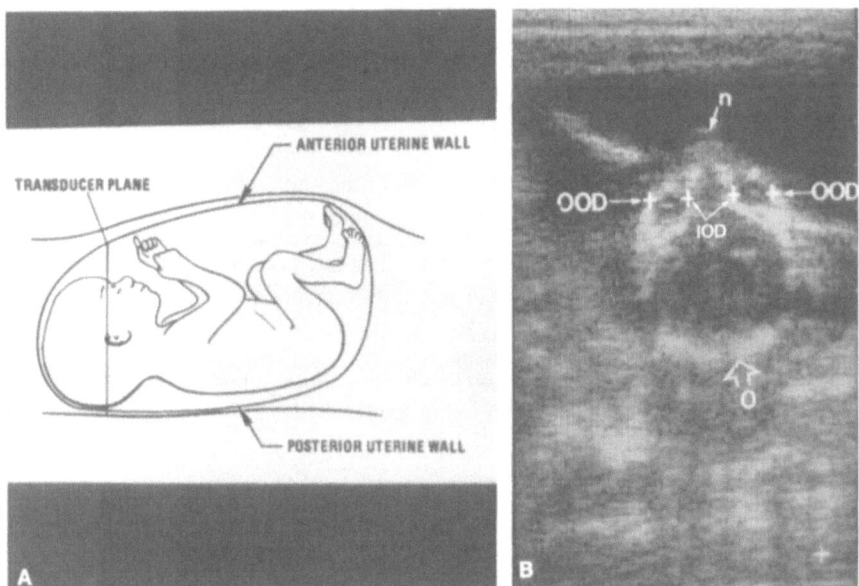

FIG. 4.2.3. FETAL ORBITS

(A) Schematic illustration demonstrating the transducer axis when obtaining the orbital distance measurements for a fetus that is in an occipital posterior position. From Mayden et al.[2]

(B) Transverse section through the fetal orbits in an occipital posterior fetal head position. The outer orbital distance (OOD) and inner orbital distance (IOD) are noted. Occiput (O), nasal bones (n). From Mayden et al.[3]

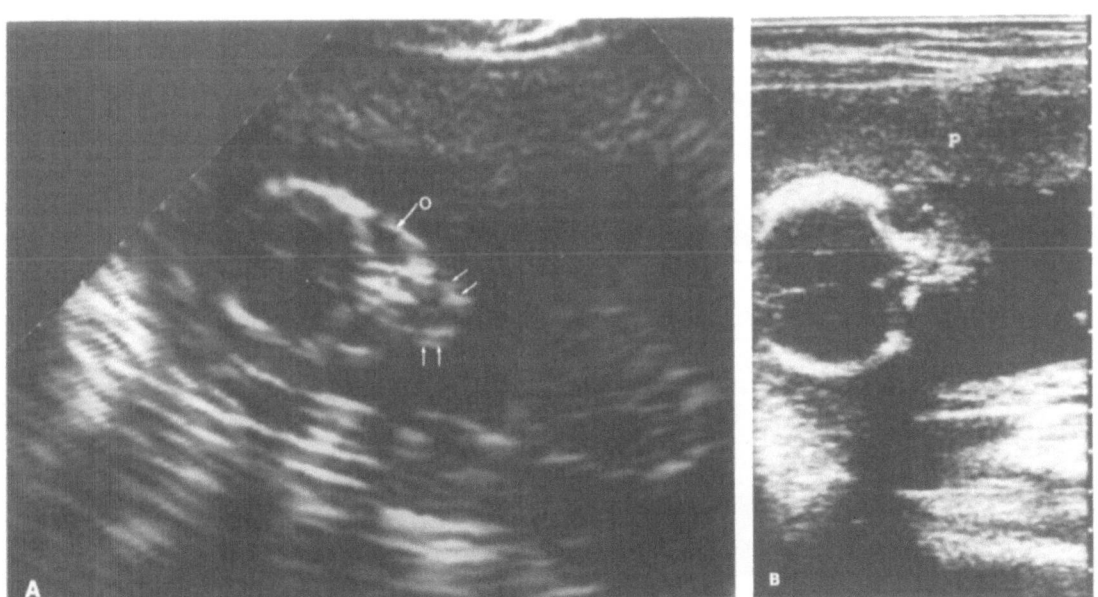

FIG. 4.2.4. THE FETAL FACE

(A) Coronal scan through the fetal face demonstrating orbit (O) and mandible (double arrows). (B) Coronal scan demonstrating the ocular lens (arrow). Placenta (P).

4.3. THE FETAL SPINE

4.3.1. The Longitudinal Axis

- Note that in the upper portion of the cervical spine a normal flaring occurs that is frequently misdiagnosed as a spinal defect.

- It is important to recognize that the two lateral borders of the spine form an almost perfect parallel line until conversion occurs in the lower sacral segment (see Fig. 4.3.1).

- Because of the flexion of the spine in pregnancy, small cervical and sacral open tube defects may be easily overlooked.

4.3.2. The Transverse View

The transverse scan should appear as a closed circle (see Fig. 4.3.2).

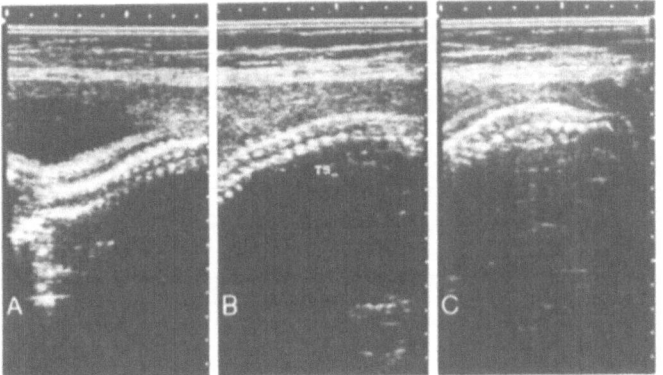

FIG. 4.3.1. FETAL SPINE: LONGITUDINAL AXIS

Longitudinal scan showing the normal fetal spine. (A) Cervical spine. (B) Thoracic spine (TS). (C) Lumbosacral spine. Normal sacral narrowing is shown (arrow.)

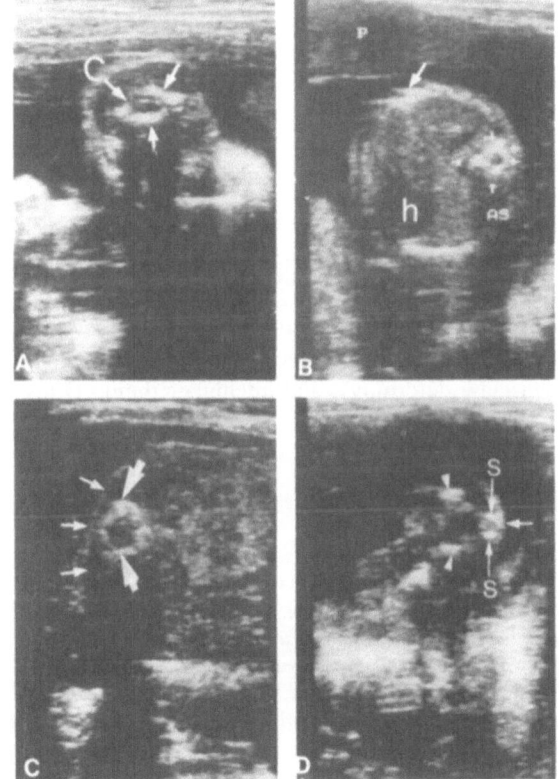

FIG. 4.3.2. FETAL SPINE: TRANSVERSE AXIS

(A)   Cervical spine (C).   (B)   Thoracic spine (small arrows), rib (large arrow), heart (h), acoustic shadowing (AS), placenta (P).   (C)   Lumbar spine (large arrows). Note the intact posterior border (small arrows) of the fetal spine.   (D)   Sacral spine (S), iliumu (arrowheads).

4.4. UPPER LIMBS

4.4.1. Humerus, Radius, and Ulna

Humerus, radius, and ulna may be used for fetal dating[6] and the antenatal diagnosis of skeletal dysplasias[7] (see Figs. 4.4.1 and 4.4.2). (For further description, see Sections 17.3 and 17.7.)

REFERENCES

6. Jeanty P, Kirkpatrick C, Dramaix-Wilmet M, et al: Ultrasonic evaluation of fetal limb growth. *Radiology* 1981;140:165.
7. Hobbins JC, Mahoney MJ: The diagnosis of skeletal dysplasias with ultrasound, in Sanders RC, James AE (eds): *The Principles and Practice of Ultrasonography in Obstetrics and Gynecology,* East Norwalk, Connecticut, Appleton-Century-Crofts, 1980, pp 191–203.

4.4.2. The Fetal Hand

High-resolution real-time equipment permits precise quantitation and assessment of fetal digits, which is of importance for the antenatal diagnosis of polydactyly, ectrodactyly (lobster-claw deformity), and hitchhiker thumb (Ellis-Van Crevald syndrome)[8-10] (see Fig. 4.4.2).

REFERENCES

8. Filly RA, Golbus MS: Ultrasonography of the normal and pathologic fetal skeleton, in Callen PW (ed): *Ultrasonography in Obstetrics and Gynecology,* Philadelphia, WB Saunders, 1983, pp 81–96.
9. Mahoney MJ, Hobbins, JC: Prenatal diagnosis of chondroectodermal dysplasia (Ellis-Van Creveld syndrome) with fetoscopy and ultrasound. *N. Engl J Med* 1977;297:258.
10. Mantagos S, Weiss RR, Mahoney MJ, et al: Prenatal diagnosis of diastrophic dwarfism. *Am J Obstet Gynecol* 1981;139:111.

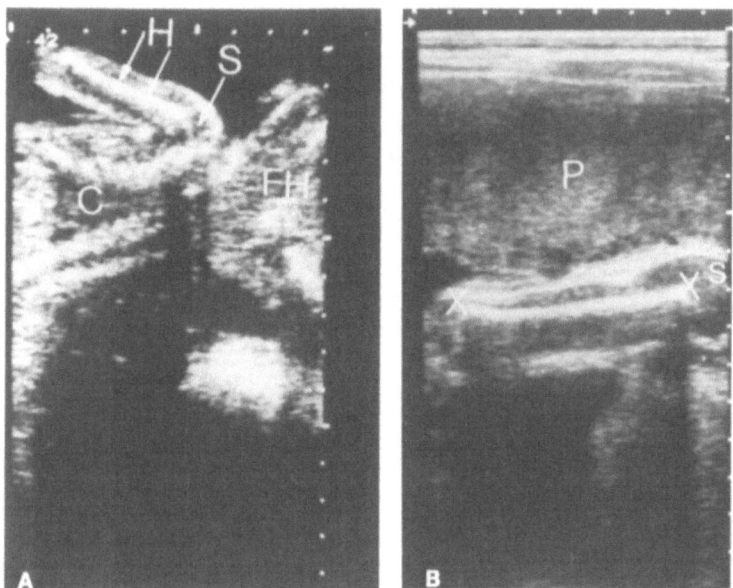

FIG. 4.4.1. THE HUMERUS

(A) Longitudinal scan of the humerus from the elbow to the shoulder(s). Fetal head (FH), chest (C), humerus (H), shoulder (S).

(B) The humerus can also be used for gestational dating (X). Placenta (P), shoulder (s).

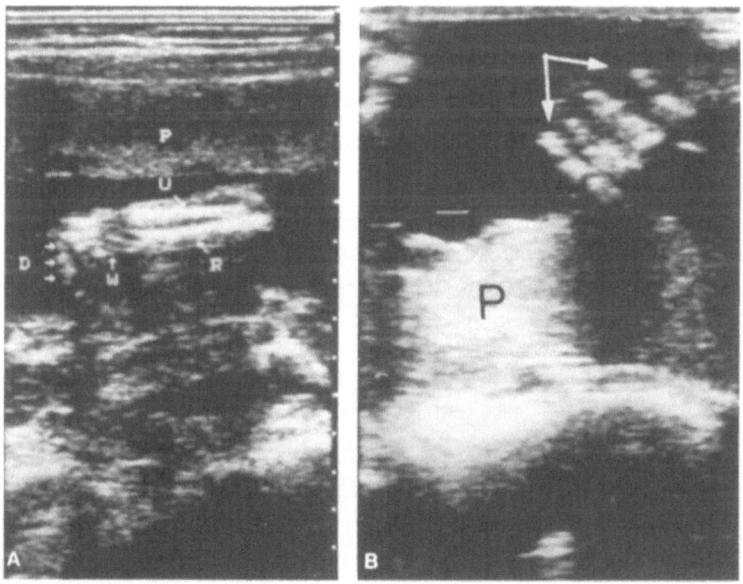

FIG. 4.4.2. FOREARM AND HAND

(A) Longitudinal scan of the fetal forearm and hand. Radius (R), ulna (U), digits (D), wrist (W), placenta (P). (B) Magnified view of the phalanges (arrows). Placenta (P).

4.5. THE FETAL THORAX

4.5.1. Fetal Ribs

Sonographically the fetal ribs are of primary importance because of the phenomenon of acoustic shadowing of bone, which may interfere with proper identification of various fetal thoracic structures lying posterior to the ribs (see Fig. 4.5.1).

4.5.2. The Fetal Lungs and Diaphragm

- Note the sonographically homogeneous appearance of the fetal lungs. The lungs are bordered laterally by the chest wall and medially by the heart. The inferior border is represented by the diaphragm (see Fig. 4.5.2).

- The fetal mediastinum has not yet been properly defined by sonographic evaluation.

- Proper sonographic identification of the fetal lungs and diaphragm is important for the antenatal diagnosis of fetal lung masses as well as structural abnormalities and diaphragmatic defects.[11,12] (See also Section 17.4.2.)

REFERENCES

11. Mayden KL, Tortora, M., Chervenak FA, et al: The antenatal sonographic detection of lung masses. *Am J Obstet Gynecol* 1984;148:349–351.
12. Harrison MR: Perinatal management of the fetus with a correctable defect, in Callen PW (ed): *Ultrasonography in Obstetrics and Gynecology*, Philadelphia, WB Saunders, 1983, pp 177–192.

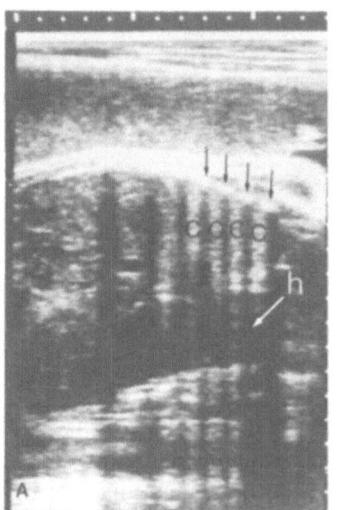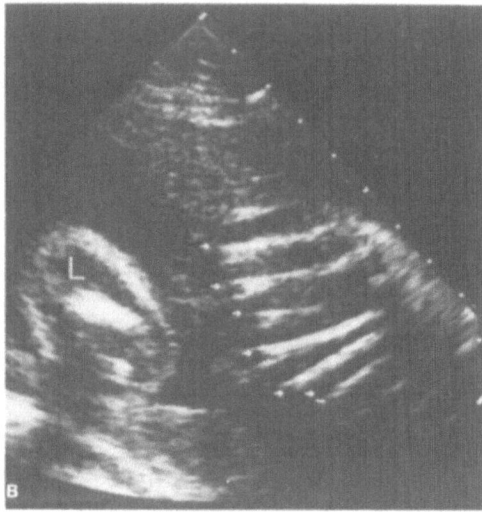

FIG. 4.5.1. THE FETAL RIBS

(A) Longitudinal scan of the fetal thorax identifying the normal appearance of the ribs (arrows) with posterior acoustic shadowing. Intercostal space (C), heart (h, white arrow).

(B) Oblique view through the fetal thorax demonstrating the entire rib (arrows). Limb (L).

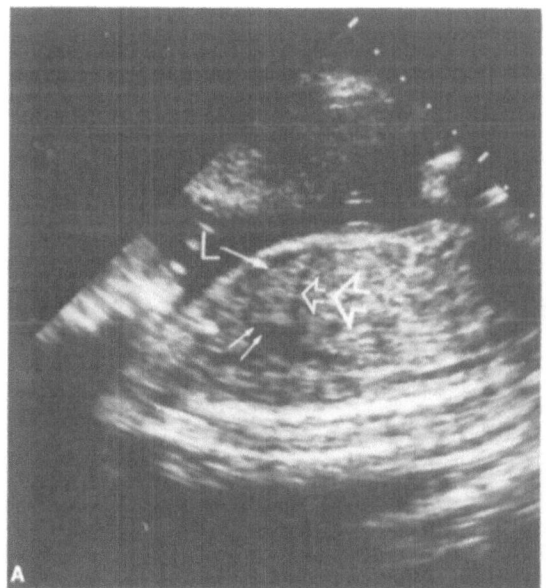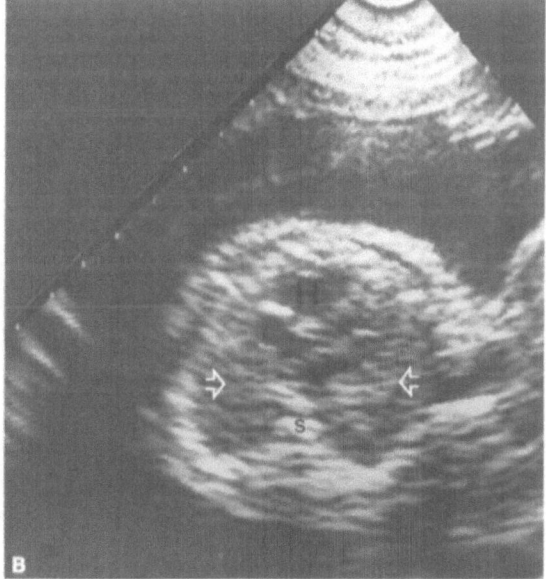

FIG. 4.5.2. THE FETAL LUNGS AND DIAPHRAGM

(A) Longitudinal scan through the fetal chest demonstrating lung tissue (L), the heart (small arrows), and the diaphragm (open arrows). Liver parenchyma can be identified inferior to the diaphragm.

(B) Transverse sector scan through the fetal chest demonstrating the fetal heart (H) and lungs (arrows). Spine (S).

CHAPTER 4 • NORMAL FETAL ANATOMY

4.6. THE FETAL HEART

- The normal anatomic position of the fetal heart in relation to the other structures within the chest represents an important reference point in ruling out chest masses, hypoplastic deformities of the lungs, and diaphragmatic hernias.[11,13]

- Identification of four chambers (see Fig. 4.6.1), the cardiac septum, and a normal heart rate of both atria and ventricles will rule out most major cardiac congenital abnormalities.[14] (See also Chapter 20 and Section 17.4.3.)

- Detailed intrauterine echocardiographic evaluation (see Fig. 4.6.2) requires considerable special expertise as well as appropriate equipment.[15] (See also Chapter 11 and Section 17.4.3.)

REFERENCES

13. Hobbins JC, Grannum PAT, Berkowitz RL, et al: Ultrasound in the diagnosis of congenital anomalies. *Am J Obstet Gynecol* 1979;134:331.
14. Sukhum P: Echocardiography and phonocardiography, in Elkayam U, Gleicher N (eds): *Cardiac Problems in Pregnancy,* New York, Alan R Liss, p 509, 1982.
15. Kerenyi TD, Gleicher N, Meller J, et al: Transplacental cardioversion of intrauterine supraventricular tachycardia. *Lancet* 1980;2:393.

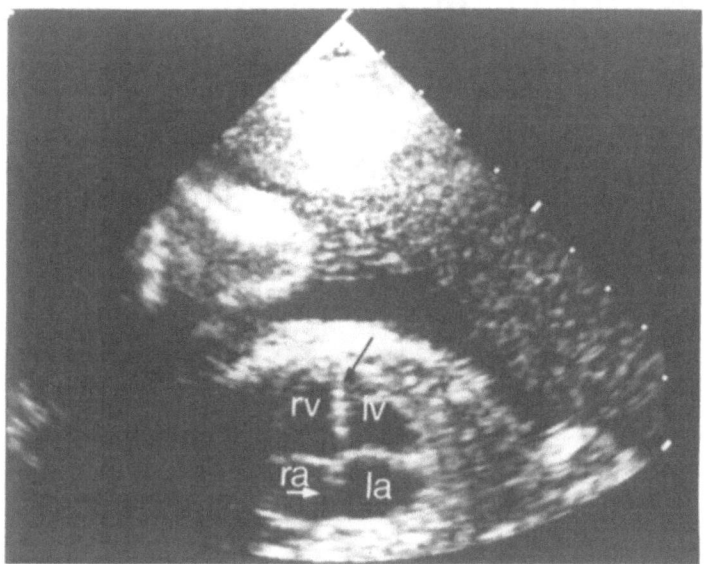

FIG. 4.6.1. FOUR-CHAMBER VIEW OF THE FETAL HEART

Transverse sector scan demonstrating the four cardiac chambers. Foramen ovale (white arrow), right ventricle (rv), left ventricle (lv), right atrium (ra), left atrium (la), intraventricular septum (black arrow).

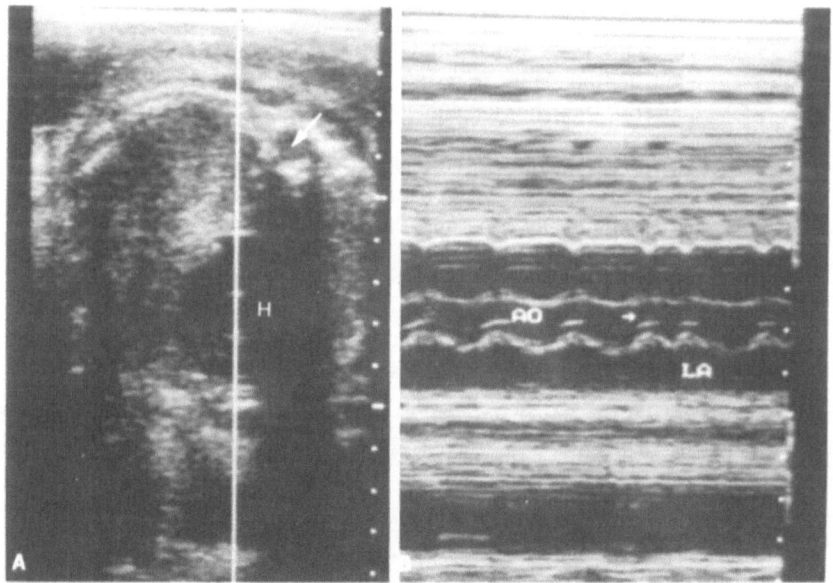

FIG. 4.6.2. INTRAUTERINE FETAL ECHOCARDIOGRAPHY

(A)   Transverse scan through the fetal heart (H) identifying the scan plane for the M-mode tracing. Spine (arrow).   (B)   M-mode tracing of the aortic root (AO), aortic valve (arrow), and left atrium (LA).

4.7. THE FETAL ABDOMEN

4.7.1. The Fetal Aorta

- Similarly to the spine, the fetal aorta can serve as a reference point in identifying the fetal position. By means of real-time sonography, pulsation of the aorta permits easy identification of this structure (see Fig. 4.7.1).

- Doppler flow studies using aortal blood flow have recently been used to calculate placental perfusion.[16]

REFERENCES

16. Campbell S, Diaz-Recasens J, Griffin DR, et al: New doppler technique for assessing uteroplacental blood flow. *Lancet* 1983;1:675.

4.7.2. The Transverse View through the Fetal Abdomen

- The borders of the normal fetal liver are difficult to visualize routinely. The acoustic impedance (density difference) between bowel and liver is minimal, and therefore their borders are difficult to appreciate sonographically.

- Recent advances in equipment permit identification of the fetal gallbladder with greater frequency. Such positive identification is important for the localization of the right hepatic lobe and the exclusion of hepatic cysts such as choledochal cysts[17,18] (see Fig. 4.7.2).

- The fetal portal system can be clearly identified and serves as a landmark for establishing appropriate abdominal circumference measurements (see Fig. 4.7.2). (For further details, see Section 7.3.)

REFERENCES

17. Chervenak FA, Berkowitz RL, Romero R, et al: The diagnosis of fetal hydrocephalus. *Am J Obstet Gynecol* 1983;6:147.
18. Elrad H, Mayden KL, Gleicher N, et al: The prenatal diagnosis of choledochal cyst. *J Ultrasound Med* 1984;4:553–555.
19. Grannum PAT, Tortora M, Mayden KL, Taylor KJW: Obsterical ultrasound, in Taylor KJW (ed): *Atlas of Ultrasonography*, ed 2. New York, Churchill Livingstone, 1985.

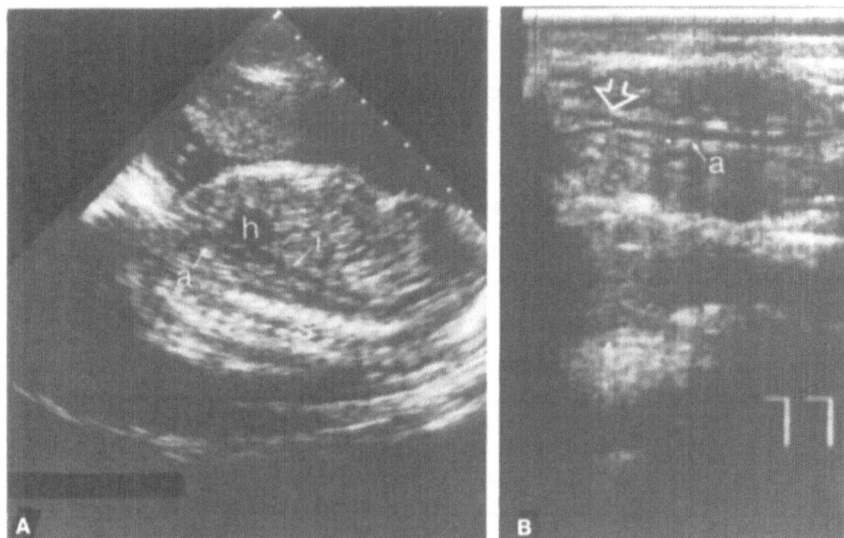

FIG. 4.7.1. THE FETAL ABDOMINAL AORTA AND OTHER MAJOR BLOOD VESSELS

(A) Longitudinal sector scan of the upper abdomen demonstrating the entrance of the inferior vena cava (I) into the heart (h). Also noted are the ascending aorta (a) and fetal spine (S).

(B) Longitudinal scan of the abdominal portion of the fetal aorta (a). The bifurcation (open arrow) into the iliac arteries is also noted.

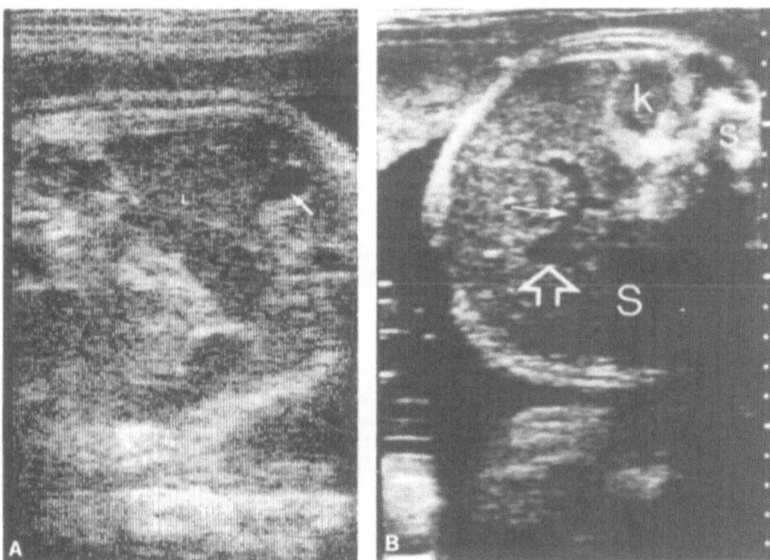

FIG. 4.7.2. FETAL ABDOMEN: TRANSVERSE AXIS

(A) Transverse scan through the fetal abdomen delineating liver (L) and the gallbladder (arrow). From Grannum *et al.*[19]

(B) Transverse scan depicting the portal venous system. Left portal vein (open arrow). Portal sinus (arrow), spine (s), stomach (S), kidney (k).

4.7.3. The Fetal Stomach

- Localization of the fetal stomach serves as a landmark for identifying the left side of the fetal abdomen, except in the situation of situs inversus (see Fig. 4.7.3).

- Visualization of a normal fetal stomach at 20 weeks gestational age supports the presence of a normal fetal swallowing mechanism.

- Failure to visualize the stomach may result from normal emptying of the stomach or fetal regurgitation. Consequently, a repeat scan after 30 min should be obtained.

- Variations in normal stomach size may be extensive. As an example, the fetal stomach may be excessively large in cases of polyhydramnios such as with maternal diabetes mellitus. (For further detail, see Chapter 9.)

- Prolonged dilatation of the stomach may indicate distal bowel obstruction such as duodenal atresia and needs further evaluation. (See also Section 17.5.2.)

- Meconium-filled bowel loops can be appreciated in the third trimester of pregnancy. Cystic dilatation, particularly when seen early in pregnancy, may indicate pathology and requires further evaluation (see Fig. 4.7.4B).

4.7.4. The Fetal Pancreas

The fetal pancreas may be visualized (see Fig. 4.7.4). While at present no clinical significance can be attached to its identification, experimental work is under way in an attempt to correlate the sonographic appearance of the pancreas with maternal diabetes mellitus.

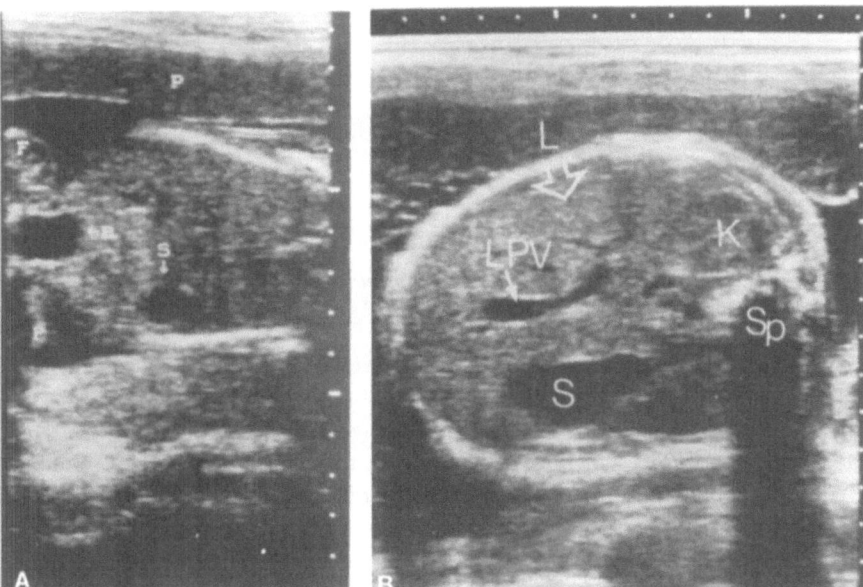

FIG. 4.7.3. THE FETAL STOMACH

(A) Longitudinal scan demonstrating the relationship of the stomach (S) to the bladder (B). Placenta (P), femur (F).

(B) Transverse scan demonstrating the normal anatomic appearance of the right-sided liver (L) and the stomach (S). Spine (Sp), left portal vein (LPV), left-sided kidney (K).

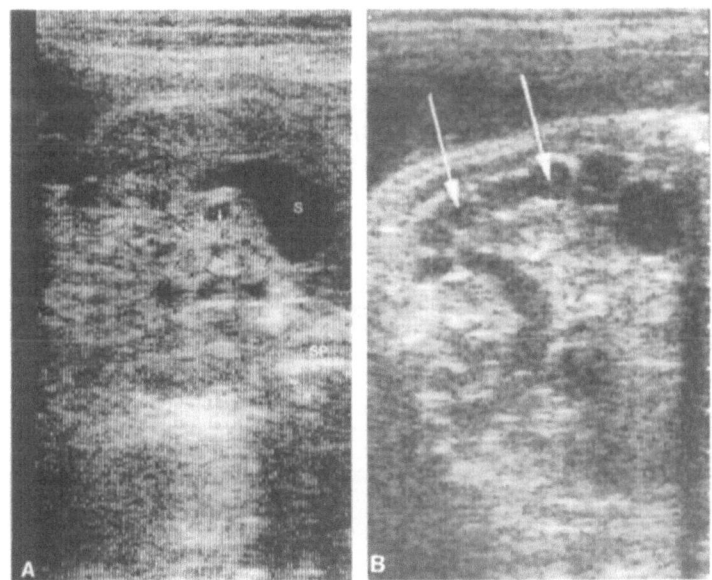

FIG. 4.7.4. THE FETAL PANCREAS AND BOWEL

(A) Transverse scan of the upper fetal abdomen demonstrating the fetal stomach (S), and pancreas (small arrows). Spine (SP). From Grannum et al.[19]

(B) Oblique view of the fetal abdomen demonstrating normal bowel loops (arrows) in the third trimester. From Grannum et al.[19]

4.8. THE FETAL URINARY TRACT

4.8.1. Fetal Kidneys and Ureters

- Because of the acoustic shadowing of the fetal spine with the fetus in a *lateral position*, the upper kidney can be more readily visualized. Manipulation of the fetus into a *back-up position* or different transducer angulations should permit identification of the opposite kidney.

- With the fetus in a *spine-up* or *spine-down position*, both kidneys can easily be identified just lateral to the fetal spine (see Fig. 4.8.1).

- Both kidney circumferences should not occupy more than one-third of the total abdominal circumference. If they occupy more than one-third of the abdomen, fetal urinary tract abnormalities have to be ruled out. (For further details, see Section 17.6.)

- It is important to identify a centrally located renal pelvis that will have the sonographic appearance of a more echo-dense area than the surrounding cortex. Minimal *caliectasis* represents a normal finding (see Fig. 4.8.2). Increased dilation, however, may be indicative of hydronephrosis and needs further evaluation. (See also Section 17.6.)

- Normal fetal ureters are difficult to define sonographically. Clear visualization of a fetal ureter may be indicative of hydroureter and requires further evaluation. (See also Section 17.6.)

- The fetal adrenals can usually be identified superior to the kidneys. Note that hypertrophy of the adrenals, particularly in conjunction with renal agenesis, can result in the false identification of adrenals for kidneys.

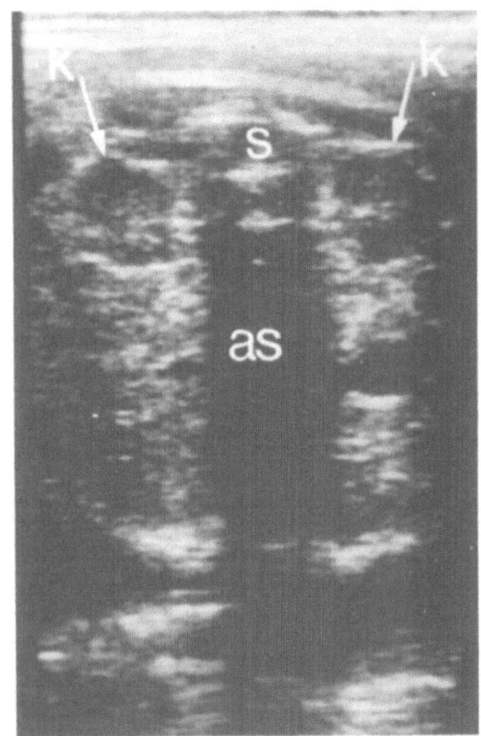

FIG. 4.8.1. LOCATION OF THE FETAL KIDNEYS

Transverse scan with the fetus in the spine-up position demonstrating the normal fetal kidneys (k) adjacent to the spine (s). Note the acoustic shadowing (as) from the spine.

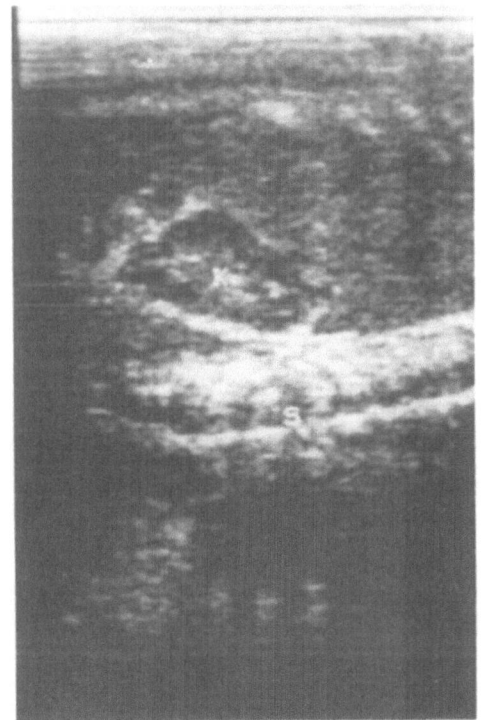

FIG. 4.8.2. NORMAL ANATOMY OF THE FETAL KIDNEY

Longitudinal scan of the fetal kidney (K) demonstrating the normal increase in echogenicity of the pelvio–caliceal complex. Spine (S).

4.8.2. The Fetal Bladder

- The bladder serves as a landmark due to its position in the pelvis. It is sonographically visible when filled with fetal urine. Visualization of the bladder therefore confirms at least unilateral renal function (see Fig. 4.8.3).

- The fetal bladder should be routinely visualized after 20 weeks gestational age.

- Absence of the fetal bladder with normal amounts of amniotic fluid may only indicate recent fetal voiding. A repeat sonogram should be obtained after 30 min. Whenever in doubt a *Lasix test* may be performed. Administration of 20–40 mg of Lasix (furosemide) to the mother will achieve a diuretic effect in the fetus. Bladder filling should be observable within 30–90 min.[20] (See also Section 17.6.2.)

- Variations in normal bladder size may be extensive. Abnormally large bladders over prolonged observation periods may indicate urethral obstruction[21] and poly-hydramnios-associated conditions. (See also Section 17.6.2.)

REFERENCES

20. Wladimiroff JW: Effect of furosemide on fetal urine production. *Br J Obstet Gynaecol* 1975;82:221.
21. Harrison MR, Filly RA, Parer JRT, et al: Management of the fetus with a urinary tract malformation. *JAMA* 1981;246:635.

4.8.3. The Fetal Urethra

The normal urethra cannot be clearly identified sonographically. Visualization of the urethra should consequently be cause for suspicion of either partial or complete urethral obstruction.

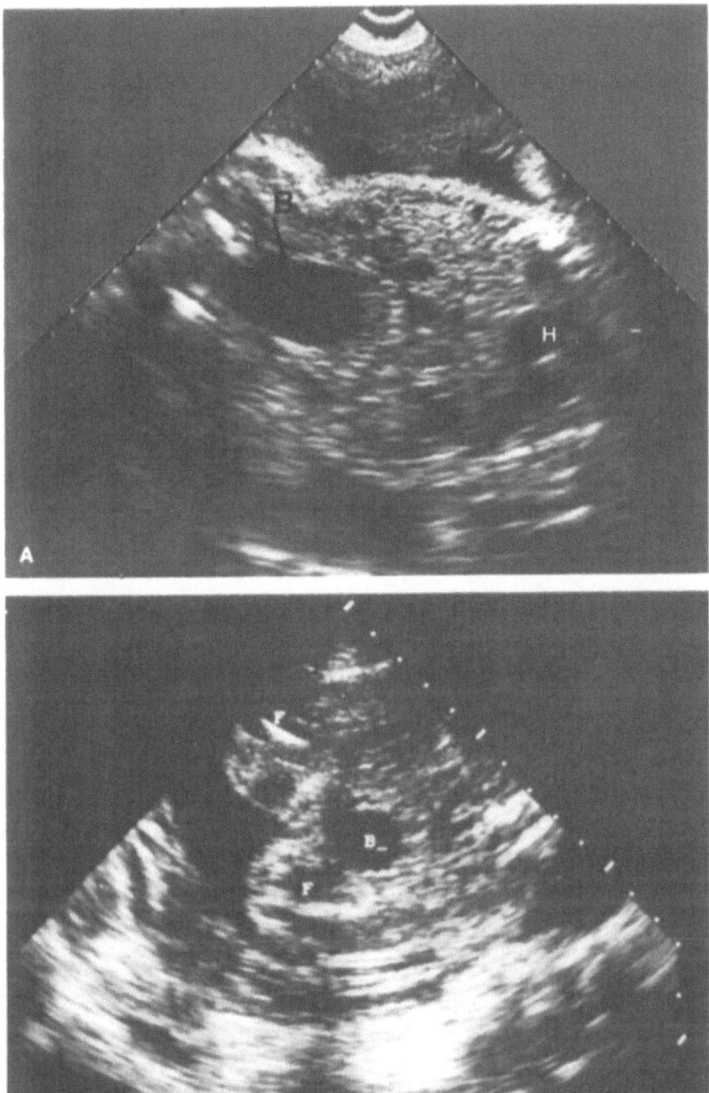

FIG. 4.8.3. THE NORMAL FETAL BLADDER

(A) Longitudinal sector scan of the fetal bladder (B) in the pelvis. Heart (H).   (B)   Transverse scan of the fetal bladder (B) and femoral heads (F).

4.9. THE FETAL GENITAL TRACT

- Sex identification through the use of sonography has recently been reported as highly accurate (more than 90%) as early as the mid-trimester of pregnancy.[22]

- Female genitalia are identified by demonstrating labia (see Fig. 4.9.1).

- Male external genitalia are identified by the demonstration of scrotum as well as penile protrusion[23] (see Fig. 4.9.2).

- Misidentification of external genitalia may occur if

  o The principal female genitalia are excessively edematous, thus mimicking a scrotum
  o The cord is thought to represent either scrotum or penile protuberance

- Excessive fluid accumulation in the scrotum (*congenital hydrocele*) can be easily diagnosed sonographically either in conjunction with a general hydrops or as an isolated generally benign lesion.

- If a cystic structure is visualized in a female fetal pelvis, the differential diagnosis of a congenital ovarian cyst or tumor, or both, has to be considered. (See Section 17.5.4.)

REFERENCES

22. Birnholz JC: Determination of fetal sex. *N Engl J Med* 1983;309:16.
23. Johnson ML, Rees GK, Hattan RA: Normal fetal anatomy, in Callen PW (ed): *Ultrasonography in Obstetrics and Gynecology*. Philadelphia, WB Saunders, 1983, pp 41–59.

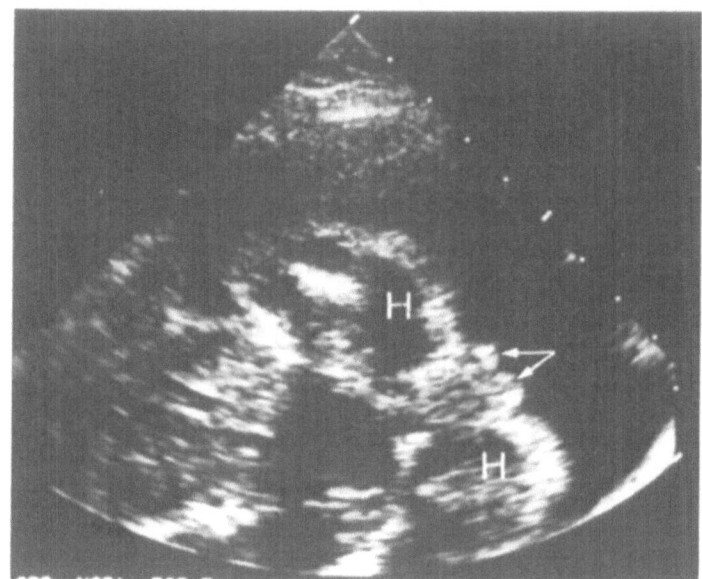

FIG. 4.9.1. FEMALE GENITALIA

Tangential view of the female genitalia (arrows). Hip (H).

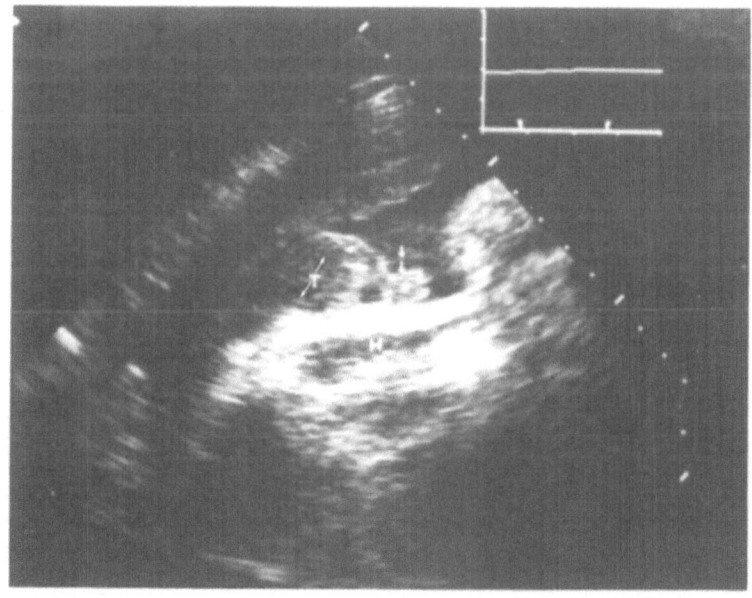

FIG. 4.9.2. MALE GENITALIA

Oblique view of the male genitalia. Penis (arrows), testes (T), hip (H).

4.10. LOWER LIMBS

4.10.1. The Femur

- The femur represents the easiest long bone to be identified (see Fig. 4.10.1). (For further details, see Sections 7.2.2, 7.3.4, and 17.7.)

- Femur length represents a standard parameter for fetal dating in the second and third trimesters of pregnancy. (See Sections 7.2.2 and 7.3.4.)

- Evaluation of femur length is also important for the antenatal detection of various forms of dwarfism.[7]

4.10.2. Tibia and Fibula

Tibia and fibula measurements are used by some investigators for gestational dating. These measurements also may be used for the prenatal diagnosis of dwarfism (see Fig. 4.10.2).

4.10.3. The Fetal Foot

Toes are more difficult to identify sonographically than are fingers. However, the antenatal diagnosis of clubfoot has been reported.[24] (See also Section 17.7.)

REFERENCE

24. Chervenak FA, Tortora M, Hobbins JC: Antenatal sonographic diagnosis of clubfoot. *J Ultrasound Med* 1985;4:49.

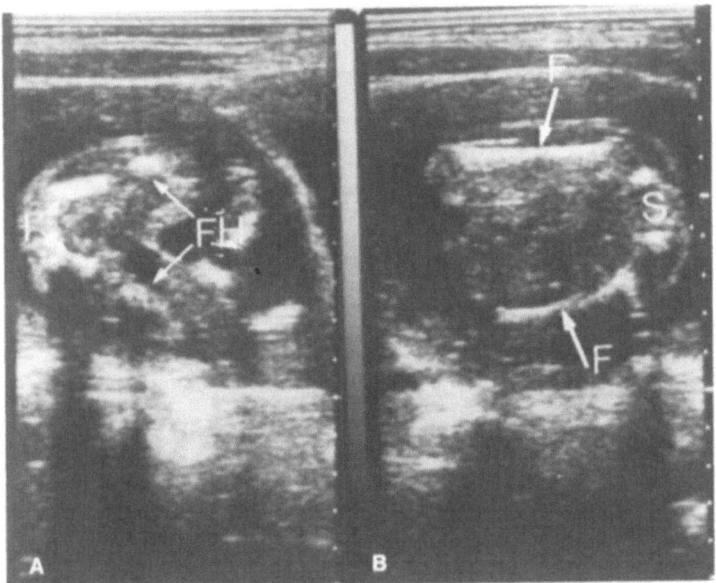

FIG. 4.10.1. THE FEMUR

(A) Cross section of the lower fetal body demonstrating the femoral heads (FH) and ilium (I).   (B) Long axis of both femurs (F). Spine (S).

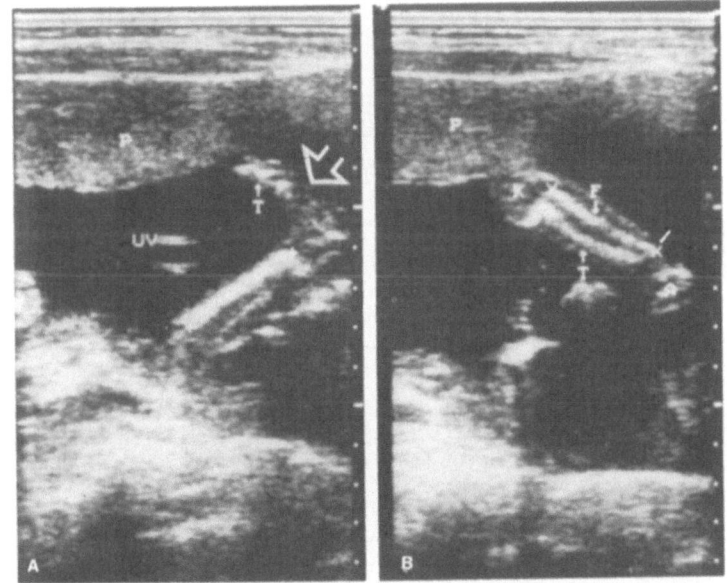

FIG. 4.10.2. LOWER LEG AND FOOT

(A) Fetal toes (T) can be visualized. Tibia (calipers), placenta (P), umbilical vein (UV), foot (open arrow).

(B) Longitudinal scan of the lower leg demonstrating the fibula (F), tibia (T), ankle (A), knee (K), and placenta (P).

Chapter 5
Cord and Placenta

5.1. THE CORD

- The normal cord contains one vein and two arteries that usually can be visualized by the latter parts of the mid-trimester (see Figs. 5.1.1 and 5.1.2).

- Recognition of a single umbilical artery should be an indication for further evaluation of the fetus to rule out associated congenital abnormalities or intra-uterine growth retardation (IUGR), or both.[1]

REFERENCE

1. Tortora M, Chervenak FA, Mayden KL, Hobbins JC: Diagnosis of single umbilical artery. *Obstet Gynecol* 1984;63:693.

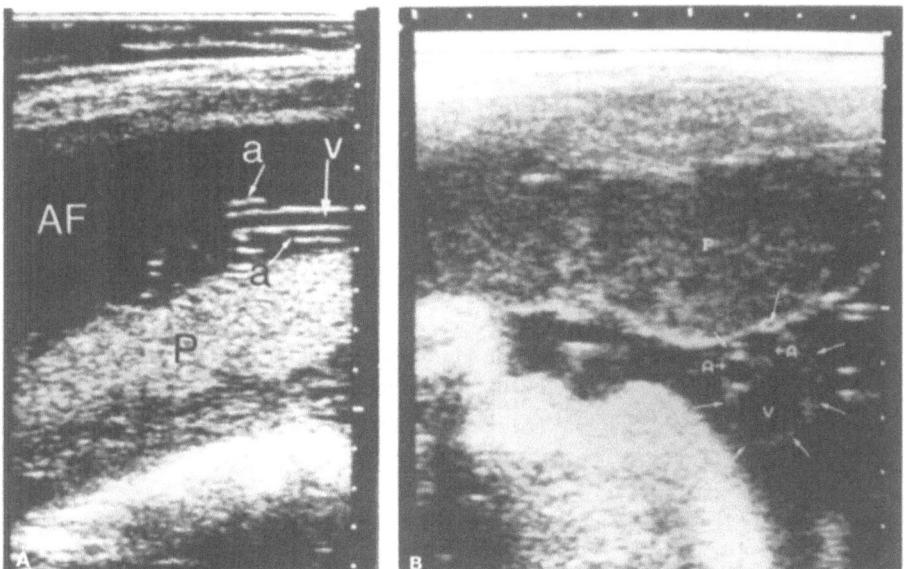

FIG. 5.1.1. THE UMBILICAL CORD

(A) Longitudinal scan of the umbilical cord demonstrating two arteries (a) and the umbilical vein (v). Placenta (P), amniotic fluid (AF).

(B) Transverse scan demonstrating the umbilical cord (arrows) visualizing two arteries (A) and the umbilical vein (V). Placenta (P).

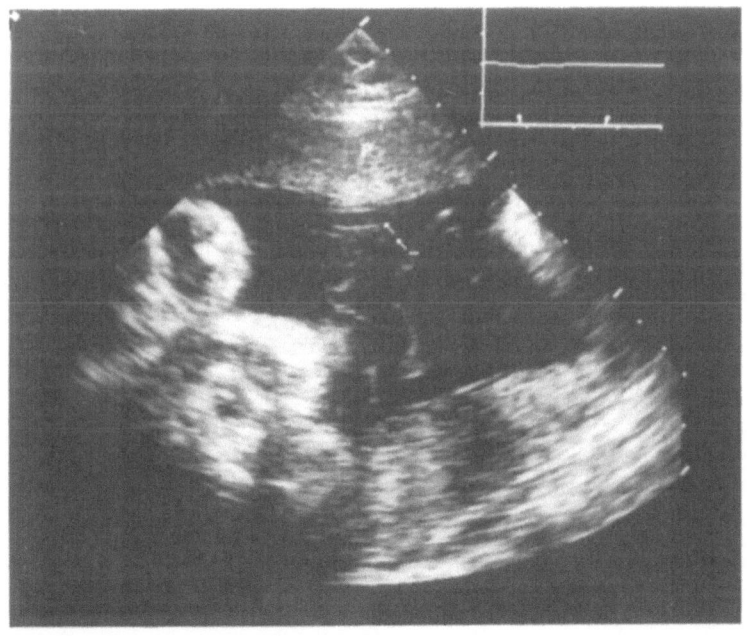

FIG. 5.1.2. PLACENTAL INSERTION OF THE FETAL CORD

Placenta (P), insertion point (arrow).

5.2. THE PLACENTA

5.2.1. General Aspects

- Unless the situation of a *threatened abortion* exists, first trimester sonography of the placenta has no specific clinically defined value. Sonographic evaluation of first trimester bleeding is discussed in Chapter 13.

- Placental sonography during the second trimester is primarily important for placental localization (see Fig. 5.2.1).

- Placental localization during the second trimester will become necessary in conjunction with genetic amniocentesis (see Chapter 6) and mid-trimester bleeding (see Chapter 16 on placenta previa and abruptio placentae).

5.2.2. Placental Anatomy

- The *chorionic plate*, whenever clearly visible, should represent an increased linear echogenic structure running uninterrupted at the fetal side of the placenta.

- The *basal plate* of the placenta should also run as an uninterrupted echogenic line. An interrupted echogenic line may be indicative of uterine activity, underlying intrauterine fibroid tumors, or placental aging. (See Section 5.2.3 on placental grading.)

- The observation of cystic clear spaces within the placenta does not always represent pathologic findings. Such areas are frequently seen at the lateral margins of the placenta and immediately beneath the chorionic plate, particularly adjacent to the cord insertion. They need to be differentiated from placental hematomas, which may occur in conjunction with placental abruption.

- Placental thickness increases with gestational age, reaching a plateau at 33 weeks, after which it decreases with increasing maturity of the placenta.

- Placental thickness does not represent an accurate diagnostic tool. However, increased thickness beyond 4.5 cm is associated with gestational diabetes, immune and nonimmune hydrops, and congenital abnormalities. A decreased thickness of the placenta is associated with preeclampsia, IUGR, severe maternal diabetes, and other severe maternal diseases.

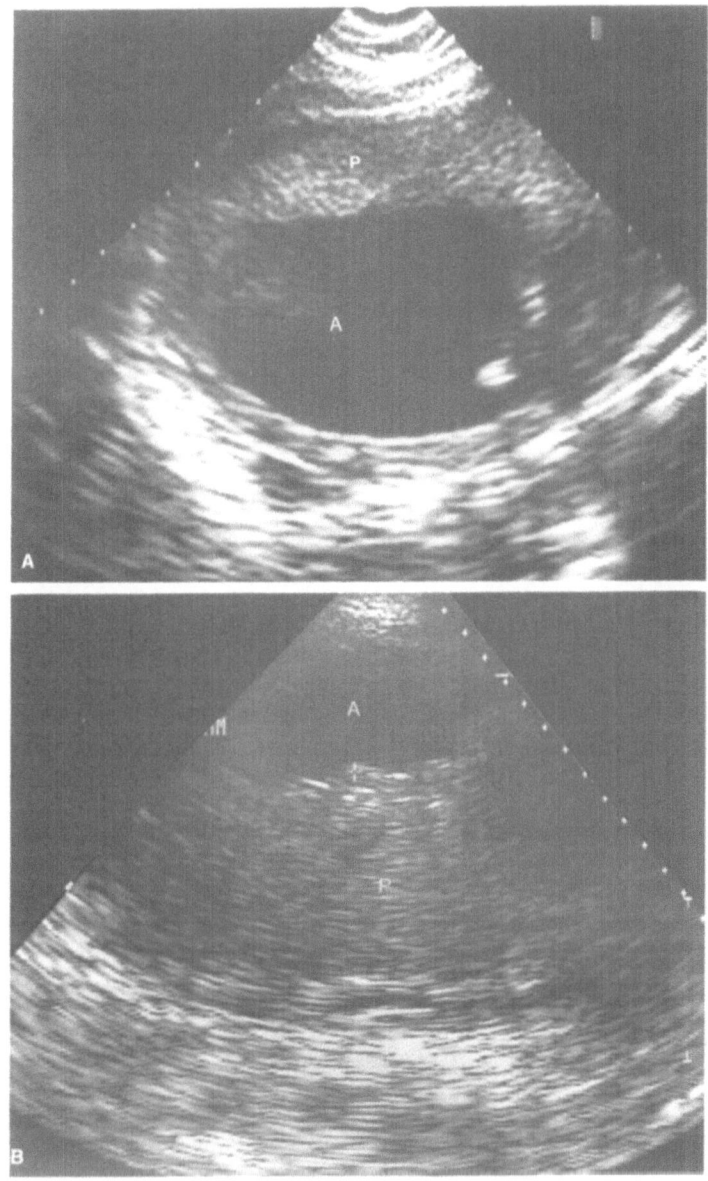

FIG. 5.2.1. PLACENTAL LOCATION

(A) Transverse sector scan at 20 weeks gestation demonstrating an anterior placenta (P). Amniotic fluid (A). (B) Transverse sector scan demonstrating a posterior placenta (P). Amniotic fluid (A).

5.2.3. Placental Grading

- Placental grading into maturity grades 0, I, II, and III has been suggested to correlate with fetal maturity status.[2] More recent work suggests that the vast majority of placentae never reach grade III. Normal pregnancies reaching a grade III placental stage probably indicate fetal maturity.

- In normal pregnancies, placental grades loosely represent the gestational ages listed in Table 5.2.1.[3]

- The sonographic picture of the various maturation grades (see Figs. 5.2.2–5.2.5) is defined as follows[2]:

Grade 0	The chorionic plate is smooth. The placenta is homogeneous in appearance without any enhanced echo-dense sonographic areas.
Grade I	The normally linear appearance of the chorionic plate may show subtle indentations. Scattered echo-dense patterns are seen throughout the placental tissue.
Grade II	Echogenic densities are seen along the basal plate and are commonly seen as commalike densities extending into the placental substance.
Grade III	Commalike densities extending from the basal plate will reach completely through the placental tissue to the chorionic plate. This process separates the placenta sonographically into cotyledons that contain an echo-free space in their center in which vascular pulsations can be seen.

TABLE 5.2.1

Placental Grade and Fetal Gestational Age[a]

Placental grade	Expected gestational age[b]
0	Up to 30 weeks gestation
I	31 weeks to term (40%)
	31 weeks to 36 weeks (45%)
II	36 weeks to term (30%)
III	At term (15–20%)

[a]Based on Grannum *et al.*[2]
[b]Incidence (%) is represented parenthetically.

- Placental gradings should be performed on the basis of the highest noted placental grade, even if that area does not represent most of the placental tissue.

- Premature maturation of the placenta before 34 weeks may indicate certain complications of pregnancy, such as IUGR, chronic hypertension, and systemic lupus erythematosus. While with normal pregnancy a grade III placenta was found to be predictive of fetal lung maturity, this was reported not to be the case in all instances of premature maturation to grade III.[2]

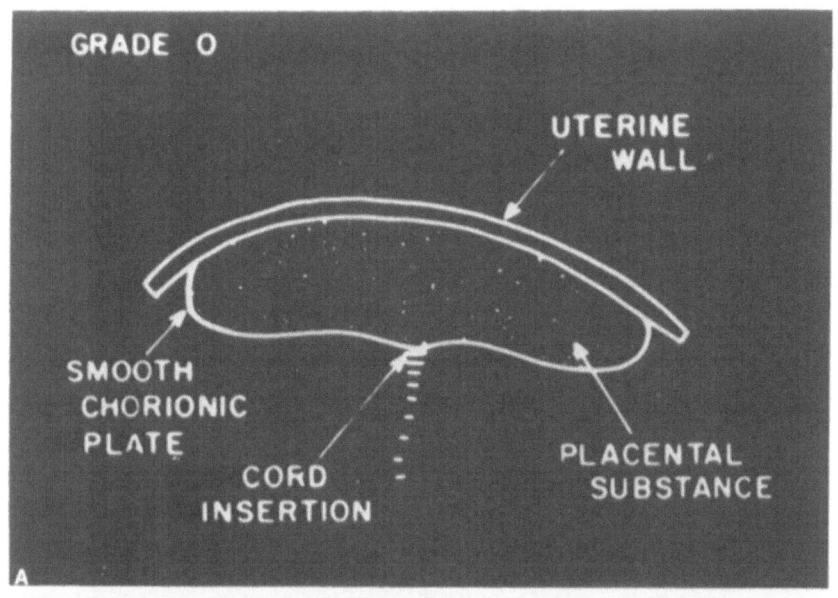

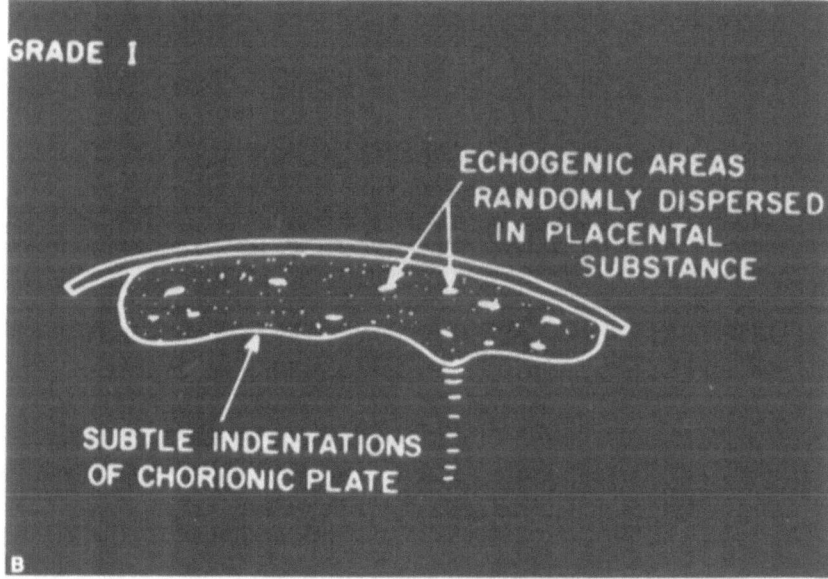

FIG. 5.2.2. SCHEMATIC DRAWINGS OF GRADES 0 AND I PLACENTAE

(A) Grade 0 placenta, anterior. From Grannum *et al.*[2]   (B) Grade I placenta, anterior. From Grannum *et al.*[2]

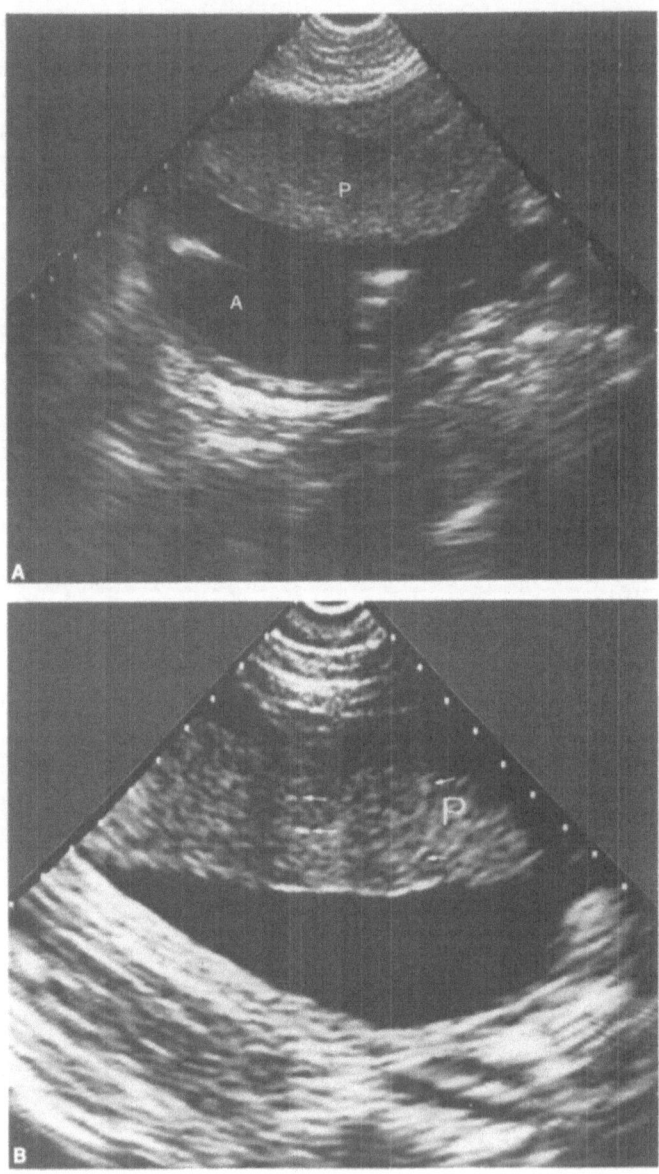

FIG. 5.2.3. GRADES 0 AND I PLACENTAE

(A)   Sector scan visualizing an anterior grade 0 placenta (P). Amniotic fluid (A).

(B)   Longitudinal scan demonstrating an anterior grade I placenta (P). Note the scattered calcifications (arrows) in the placental tissue.

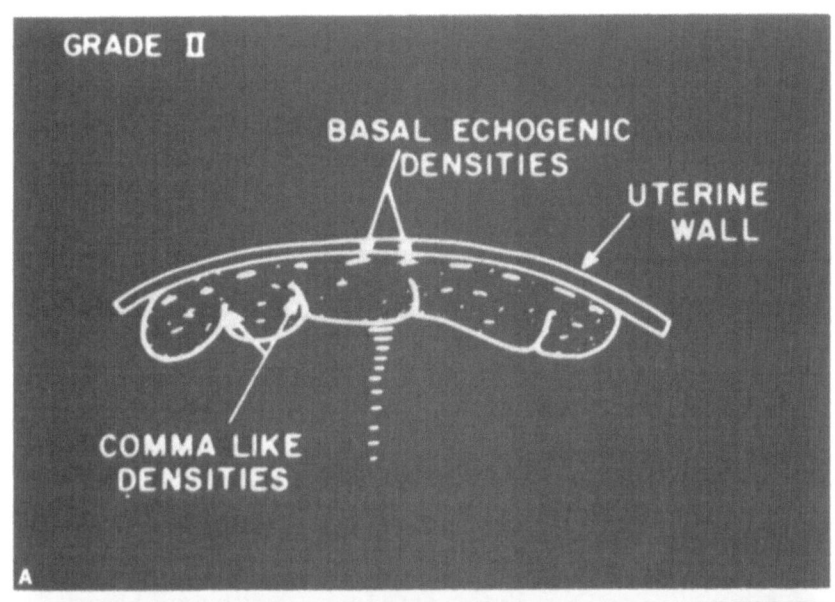

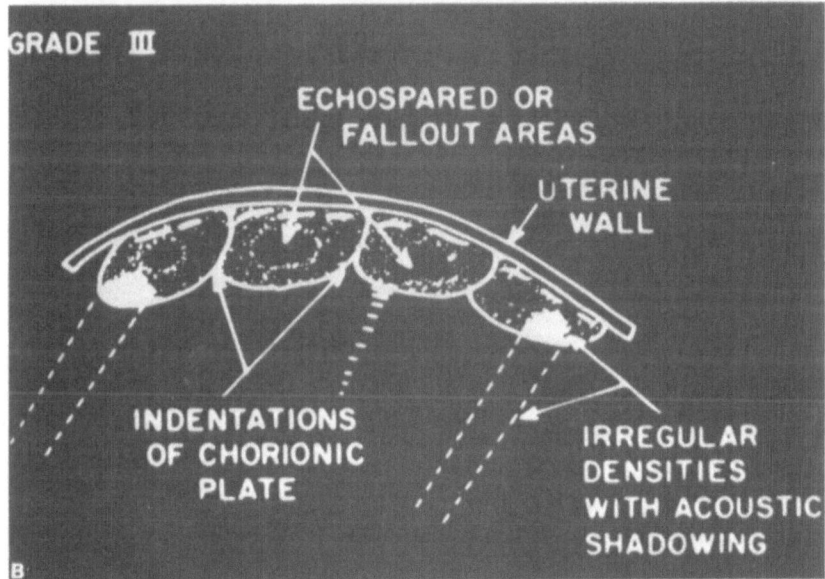

FIG. 5.2.4. SCHEMATIC DRAWING OF GRADES II AND III PLACENTAE

(A) Grade II placenta, anterior. From Grannum *et al.*[2] (B) Grade III placenta, anterior. From Grannum *et al.*[2]

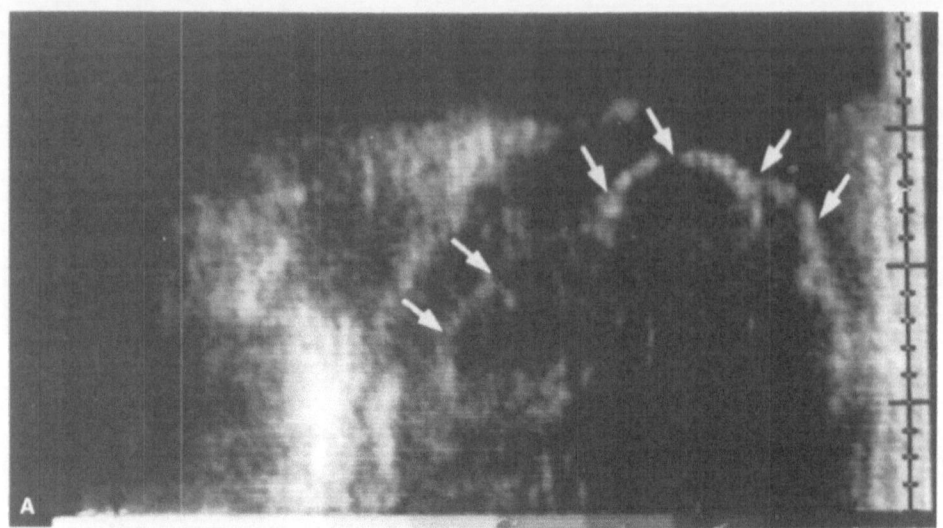

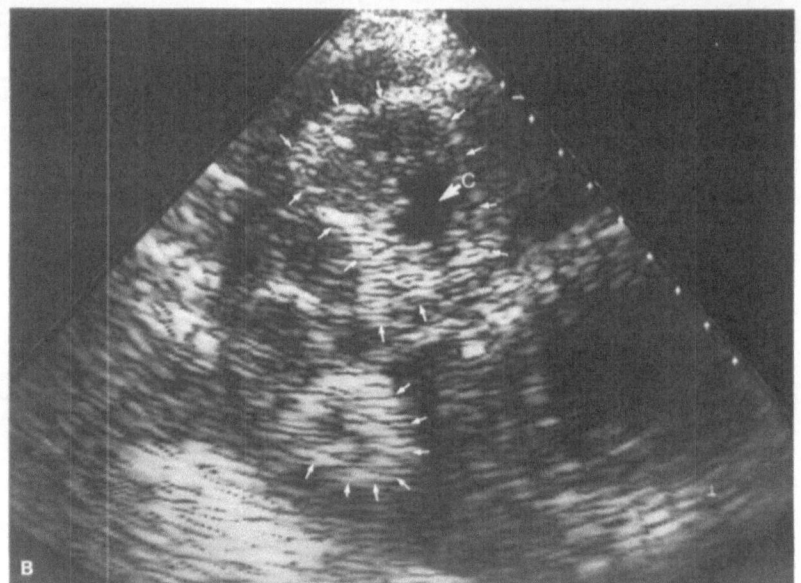

FIG. 5.2.5. GRADES II AND III PLACENTAE

(A) Sonographic demonstration of a grade II placenta. Note that the calcifications are not completely surrounding the cotyledons (arrows).

(B) Transverse sector scan through the uterine fundus demonstrating a grade III placenta. Note the echo-spared center of the cotyledon (C) and the calcifications extending from the chorionic to basal plate (small arrows).

REFERENCES

2. Grannum PAT, Berkowitz RL, Hobbins JC: The ultrasonic changes in the maturing placenta and their relation to fetal pulmonic maturity. *Am J Obstet Gynecol* 1979;133:915.

3. Grannum PAT, Hobbins JC: The placenta, in Callen PW (ed): *Ultrasonography in Obstetrics and Gynecology*. Philadelphia, WB Saunders, 1983, p 141.

Chapter 6
Amniocentesis

Amniocentesis has been greatly enhanced by the use of ultrasound. Ultrasound can provide an assessment of fetal anatomy and growth and also permits the correct placement of the needle into the amniotic cavity.

- Genetic mid-trimester amniocentesis is best performed at 16–18 weeks gestational age (see Fig. 6.1.1).

- Sonographic localization of the placenta as well as sonographic control of the amniocentesis process itself have recently been recommended[1] (see Fig. 6.1.2).

- The placenta should be avoided. However, with anterior wall placentae, when no window can be visualized, the placenta may be crossed using a 22-gauge aspiration needle, as long as care is taken to avoid the area of cord insertion.

- Fetal parts should be identified before amniocentesis to prevent fetal trauma from the needle.

- If sonography is performed for amniocentesis, a routine sonographic evaluation of the pregnancy should be performed before the procedure in order to achieve accurate dating, rule out multiple pregnancies, and detect any gross malformations.

- All Rh-negative patients undergoing amniocentesis must receive anti-D immunoglobulin.

- Fetal heart rate activity should be reconfirmed after amniocentesis.

- In the third trimester amniocentesis, amniotic fluid may be decreased, requiring suprapubic taps.

REFERENCES

1. Jeanty P, Rodesch F, Romero R, et al: How to improve your amniocentesis technique. *Am J Obstet Gynecol* 1983;146:593.
2. Platt LD, DeVore GR, Gimovski ML: Failed amniocentesis: The role of membrane tenting. *Am J Obstet Gynecol* 1983;144:479.

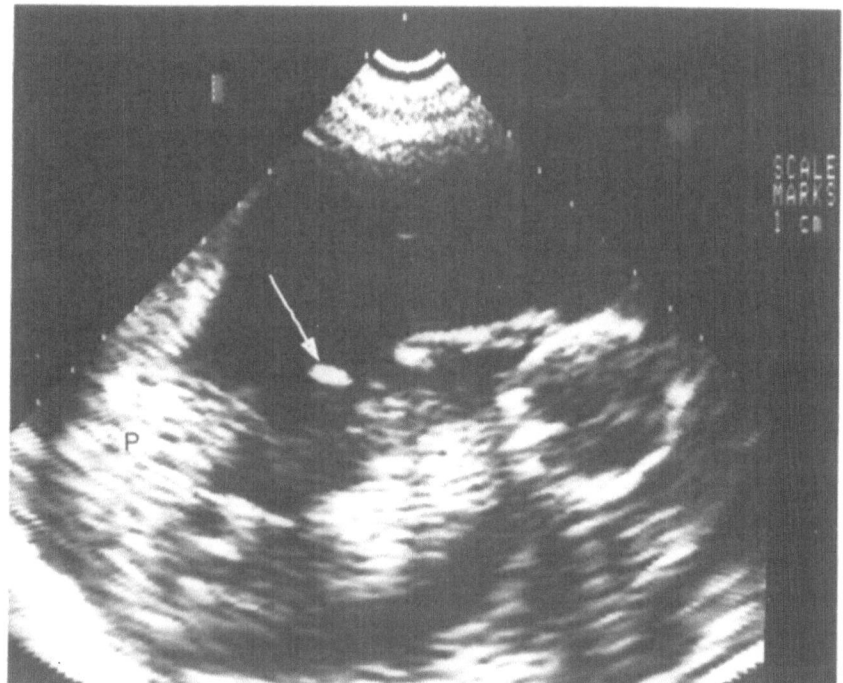

FIG. 6.1.1. SECOND TRIMESTER AMNIOCENTESIS

Longitudinal scan demonstrating the needle track (arrow) in the amniotic fluid during a second trimester amniocentesis. Placenta (P).

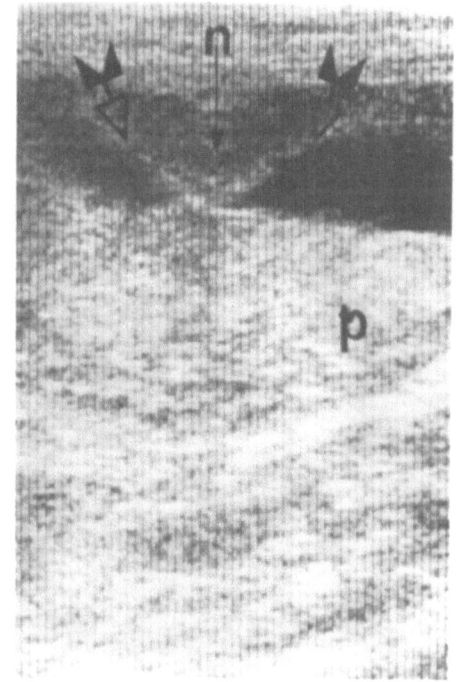

FIG. 6.1.2. TENTING OF MEMBRANES DURING AMNIOCENTESIS

Membranes can be seen to project into the amniotic cavity (arrow), preceding the needle tip (n). The placenta (p) is posterior. From Platt *et al.*[2]

Chapter 7
Gestational Dating

7.1. FIRST TRIMESTER DATING

- Sonographic estimation of gestational age is based on the last normal menstrual period (LNMP)—*not* the date of conception.

- Gestational dating during the first trimester is based on the following parameters:

4–6 weeks	Identification of a gestational sac without internal echoes (see Fig. 7.1.1)
5–7 weeks	Appearance of internal echoes (fetal pole/yolk sac)
6–7 weeks	Identification of fetal cardiac activity
7–9 weeks	Identification of longitudinal axis of the fetus; ability to obtain crown–rump length (CRL)
7–12 weeks	Measurement of crown–rump length (see Fig. 7.1.2)

- Gestational age can be assessed by crown–rump length,[1] as shown in Table 7.1.1.

- Among all available single-measurement dating methods, the crown–rump length is the most accurate, with an error of only ±5 days. When three crown-rump lengths are averaged the accuracy improves to ± 3 days.[1]

- Crown–rump length is obtained by measuring the longest axis of the fetus, not including the cord or yolk sac.

REFERENCE

1. Robinson HP, Fleming JE: A critical evaluation of sonar ''crown rump length'' measurements. *Br J Obstet Gynaecol* 1975;82:702.

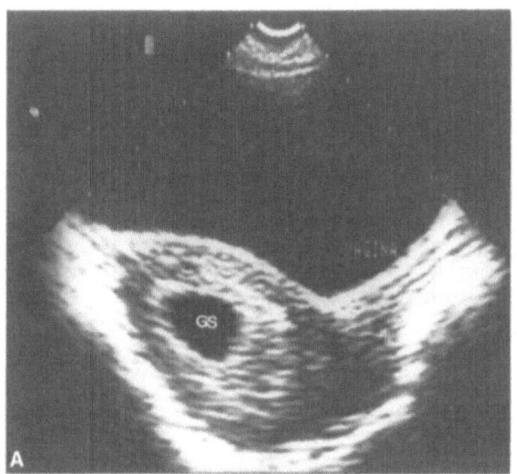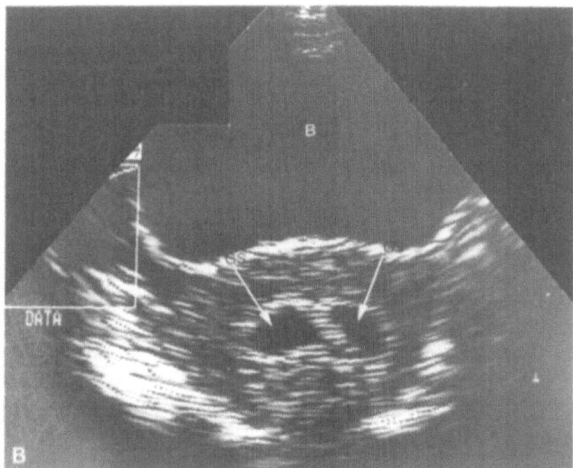

FIG. 7.1.1.   NORMAL GESTATIONAL SACS: 4–6 WEEKS

(A)   Longitudinal sector scan of a singleton gestational sac with no internal echoes. Note the smooth and thickened rindlike appearance of the sac outlined with the uterine echoes. Gestational sac (GS).

(B)   Normal twin gestational sacs with no internal echoes and membrane separating the sacs. Gestational sac (GS), bladder (B).

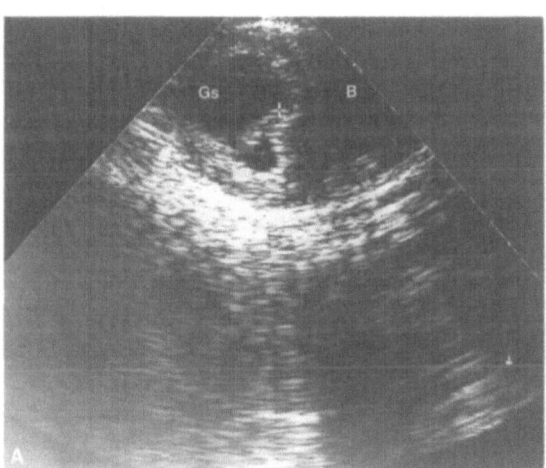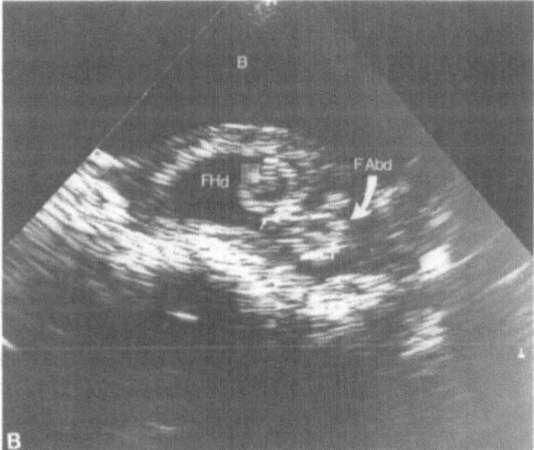

FIG. 7.1.2.   CROWN–RUMP LENGTH (CRL)

(A)   CRL at 7–8 weeks gestational age. Gestational sac (GS), bladder (B).

(B)   CRL at 10–11 weeks gestational age. Small arrow indicates fetal orbit. Gestational sac (GS), bladder (B), fetal head (FHd), fetal abdomen (FAbd).

TABLE 7.1.1

Assessment of Gestational Age in the First Trimester by Crown–Rump Length[a]

CRL (mm)	−2 SD	Mean weeks	+2 SD	CRL (mm)	−2 SD	Mean weeks	+2 SD
7		6.25	7.15	39	10	10.65	11.35
8		6.45	7.3	40	10.1	10.75	11.45
9		6.7	7.55	41	10.2	10.8	11.55
10	6.25	6.9	7.7	42	10.3	10.9	11.65
11	6.5	7.1	7.9	43	10.4	11.05	11.7
12	6.6	7.25	8.1	44	10.45	11.1	11.8
13	6.85	7.45	8.25	45	10.55	11.2	11.9
14	7.00	7.60	8.45	46	10.66	11.3	12
15	7.15	7.75	8.60	47	10.7	11.35	12.05
16	7.3	7.9	8.70	48	10.8	11.45	12.15
17	7.45	8.1	8.9	49	10.9	11.55	12.25
18	7.60	8.2	9.0	50	10.95	11.6	12.3
19	7.75	8.4	9.15	51	11.1	11.7	12.4
20	7.9	8.5	9.3	52	11.15	11.8	12.5
21	8.05	8.6	9.4	53	11.2	11.85	12.55
22	8.15	8.8	9.55	54	11.3	11.95	12.65
23	8.3	8.9	9.65	55	11.4	12.05	12.75
24	8.4	9.05	9.8	56	11.5	12.1	12.8
25	8.55	9.15	9.9	57	11.55	12.2	12.9
26	8.7	9.3	10	58	11.65	12.3	12.95
27	8.8	9.4	10.1	59	11.7	12.35	13.05
28	8.9	9.5	10.25	60	11.8	12.45	13.15
29	9.05	9.65	10.35	61	11.85	12.5	13.2
30	9.15	9.7	10.45	62	11.9	12.6	13.3
31	9.25	9.85	10.55	63	12	12.65	13.4
32	9.35	9.95	10.65	64	12.05	12.75	13.45
33	9.45	10.05	10.75	65	12.1	12.85	13.55
34	9.55	10.15	10.85	66	12.2	12.9	13.6
35	9.6	10.2	10.95	67	12.3	12.95	13.7
36	9.7	10.35	11.05	68	12.35	13.05	13.75
37	9.8	10.4	11.15	69	12.45	13.1	13.8
38	9.9	10.55	11.25	70	12.5	13.15	13.9

[a]From Robinson.[1]

7.2. SECOND TRIMESTER DATING

- Crown–rump length becomes an inaccurate indicator of gestational age after 12–13 weeks because of significant spinal flexion.

- Gestational dating during the second trimester, gestational weeks 12–30, is best based on fetal biparietal diameter (BPD) measurements.[2] More recently, femur length has been established as a reliable second dating parameter.[3]

- Assessment of gestational age is established by fetal BPD (see Section 7.2.1) and femur length.[2,3]

- Femur length can be predicted at various points in gestation.[4] Table 7.2.1 compares the femur length correlations arrived at by several investigators.

TABLE 7.2.1

Comparison of Predicted Femur Lengths at Points in Gestation[a]

Menstrual age (weeks)	Femur length (mm)			
	Filly et al. (1981)[2][b]	Jeanty et al. (1981)[4][c]	Hadlock et al. (1982)[3][b]	Hadlock et al. (1982)[3][c]
12	—	09	14	08
13	—	12	12	11
14	16	16	19	15
15	19	19	21	18
16	22	23	23	21
17	25	26	26	24
18	28	30	28	27
19	32	33	30	30
20	35	36	33	33
21	38	39	35	36
22	41	42	38	39
23	44	45	40	42
24	47	48	42	44
25	50	51	45	47
26	53	54	47	49
27	55	57	49	52
28	57	59	52	54
29	61	62	54	56
30	63	65	57	58
31	—	67	59	61
32	—	70	61	63
33	—	72	64	65
34	—	74	66	66
35	—	77	69	68
36	—	79	71	70
37	—	81	73	72
38	—	83	76	73
39	—	85	78	75
40	—	87	80	76

[a]From Callen, p. 273.[5] See also specific studies cited (refs. 2, 3, and 4).
[b]Linear function.
[c]Linear quadratic function.

REFERENCES

2. Filly RA, Golbus MS, Carey JC, et al: Short-limbed dwarfism: Ultrasonographic diagnosis by mensuration of fetal femoral length. *Radiology* 1981;138:653.
3. Hadlock FP, Harrist RB, Deter RL, et al: Fetal femur length as a predictor of menstrual age: Sonographically measured. *AJR* 1982;138:875.
4. Jeanty P, Kirkpatrick C, Dramaix-Wilmet, et al: Ultrasonic evaluation of fetal limb growth. *Radiology* 1981;140:165.
5. Callen PW (ed): *Ultrasonography in Obstetrics and Gynecology.* Philadelphia, WB Saunders, 1983.

7.2.1. Biparietal Diameter

- Parameters for an adequate fetal BPD are as follows:

  o The level of BPD should be obtained below the level of the lateral ventricles and just above the level of the orbits and cerebral peduncles. (See Section 4.2, for further details.)

  o The shape of BPD should be oval.

  o Midline should be equidistant from both lateral borders.

  o The level of BPD should include the thalamus, the cavuum septum pellucidum, and the pulsations of the middle cerebral artery (sylvian fissure or insula).

  o Depending on the standard table used, BPD measurements may go from outer to inner or from outer to outer skull edges. Table 7.2.2 uses outer to inner measurements.

  o All BPD measurements should be obtained perpendicular to the midline (see Figs. 7.2.1–7.2.4).

- The standard error in gestational age using a single mid-trimester BPD measurement is 1–1.5 weeks at 12–20 weeks and increases to 1.5–2 weeks at 20–30 weeks.

- At times BPD cannot be properly obtained as in straight occipital anterior or occipital posterior positions of the fetal head. In such circumstances, other parameters such as femur length have to be relied on.

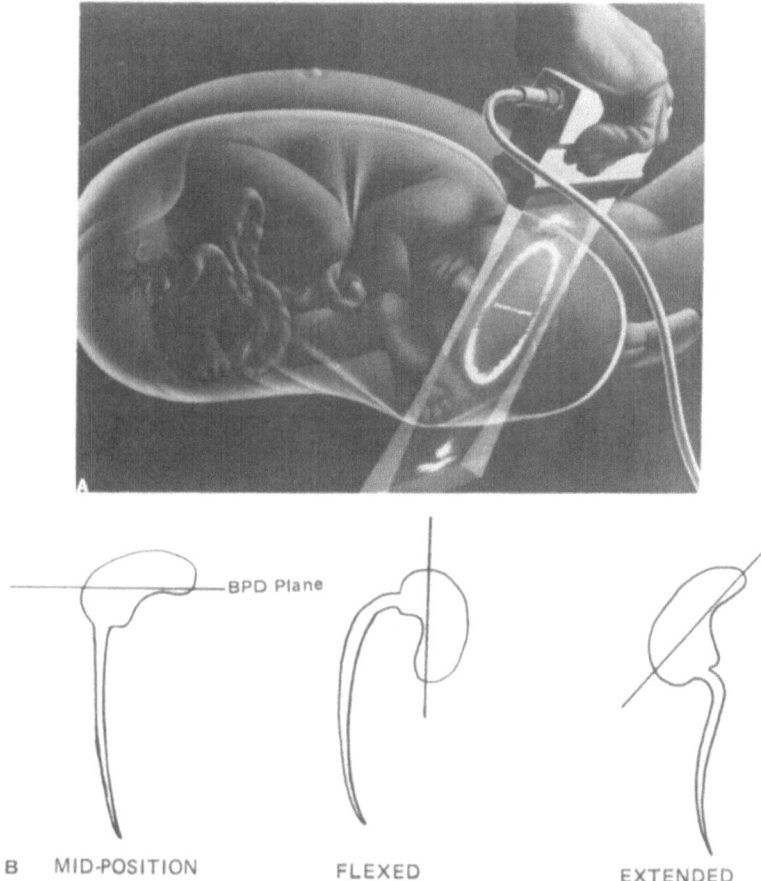

BPD Plane

B   MID-POSITION   FLEXED   EXTENDED

FIG. 7.2.1.   GRAPHIC SCHEME ON HOW TO OBTAIN A FETAL BIPARIETAL DIAMETER

(A)   Schematic illustration of the level of the BPD with the fetal head in an occipital transverse position. (Reproduced with permission from Advanced Diagnostic Research, Tempe, Arizona.)

(B)   Schematic representation of the BPD plane with the fetal head in the mid, flexed, and extended position. BPD plane should be perpendicular to the entrance of the cervical spine into the head. (Illustrations by R. V. Giglia.)

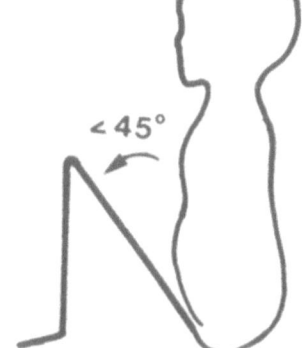

FIG. 7.2.2.   GRAPHIC SCHEME ON HOW TO OBTAIN A FEMUR LENGTH

Schematic illustration of the femoral angle with the fetus in a fetal position. Femurs can be visualized by angling 45°–90° from the long axis of the fetal body.

From Sabbagha, p. 226.[10]

TABLE 7.2.2
Correlation of Predicted Menstrual Age Based on Fetal Biparietal Diameters[a]

Menstrual age (weeks)	BPD mean values (mm)					
	Composite Sabbagha and Hughey (1978)[6]	Composite Kurtz et al. (1980)[7]	Kurtz et al. (1980)[7]	Kurtz et al. (1980)[7]	Hadlock et al. (1982)[8]	Shepard and Filly (1982)[9]
14	28	27	28	26	27	28
15	32	31	31	29	30	31
16	36	34	35	33	33	34
17	39	38	39	36	37	37
18	42	41	42	40	40	40
19	45	45	46	43	43	43
20	48	48	49	46	46	46
21	51	51	52	50	50	49
22	54	54	55	53	53	52
23	58	57	58	56	56	55
24	61	60	61	59	58	57
25	64	63	64	61	61	60
26	67	66	67	64	64	63
27	70	69	69	67	67	65
28	72	71	72	70	70	68
29	75	74	75	72	72	71
30	78	76	77	75	75	73
31	80	79	79	77	77	76
32	82	81	81	79	79	78
33	85	83	83	82	82	80
34	87	85	85	84	84	83
35	88	87	87	86	86	85
36	90	89	89	88	88	88
37	92	91	91	90	90	90
38	93	92	92	92	91	92
39	94	94	94	94	93	95
40	95	95	95	95	95	97

[a]From Callen, p. 326.[5] See also specific studies cited (refs. 6, 7, 8, 9).

REFERENCES

6. Sabbagha RE, Hughey M: Standardization of sonar cephalometry and gestational age. *Obstet Gynecol* 1978;52:402.
7. Kurtz AB, Wapner RJ, Kurtz RJ, et al: Analysis of biparietal diameter as an accurate indicator of gestational age. *J Clin Ultrasound* 1980;8:319.
8. Hadlock FP, Deter RL, Harrist RB, et al: Fetal biparietal diameter: A critical reevaluation of the relation to menstrual age by means of real-time ultrasound. *J Ultrasound Med* 1982;1:97–104.
9. Shepard M, Filly RA: A standardized plane for biparietal diameter measurement. *J Ultrasound Med* 1982;1:145.
10. Sabbagha RE: *Diagnostic Ultrasound Applied to Obstetrics and Gynecology*. Hagerstown, Md, Harper & Row, 1980.

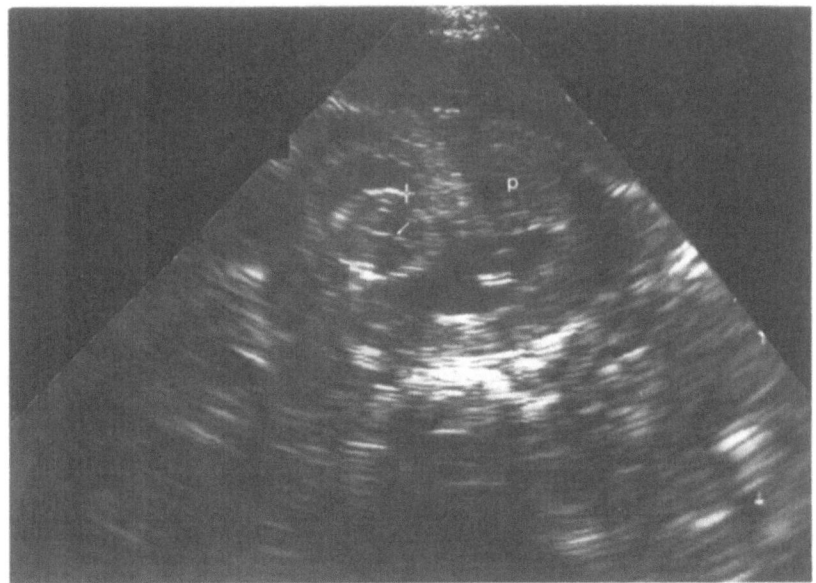

FIG. 7.2.3. LANDMARKS FOR BIPARIETAL DIAMETER: 13 WEEKS

Transverse sector scan through the fetal head at the level of the BPD. Note the equidistant midline (arrow) and oval shape. Placenta (p).

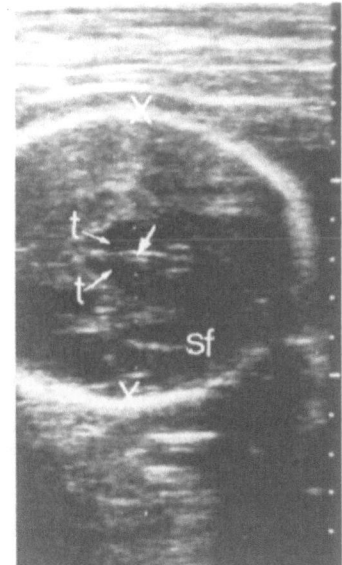

FIG. 7.2.4. LANDMARKS FOR BIPARIETAL DIAMETER: 30–32 WEEKS

Transverse scan through the fetal head at the level of the BPD. Identification of the thalami (t), 3rd ventricle (arrow), and sylvian fissure (sf) serve as landmarks for an accurate measurement (X).

7.2.2. Femur Length

- Parameters for establishing accurate femur lengths are as follows:
  - The longest axis of the femur should be measured, not including the femoral head.
  - Measurement should be obtained from the distal end of the shaft to the greater trochanter (see Figs. 7.2.2. and 7.2.5).
  - The acoustic shadowing of the femur aids in proper measurement (see Fig. 7.2.5).

- The standard error in gestational age using a single mid-trimester femur length evaluation was reported at a level approximately equal to that of the BPD.[11]

7.2.3. Other Parameters Used in Mid-Trimester

- Measurements of fetal orbital diameter[12] (see Fig. 7.2.6 and Table 7.3.2) and of long bones other than the femur[13] have been used by some investigators as a means of evaluating gestational age during the mid-trimester.

- These parameters are increasingly used as further adjuncts in assessing fetal gestational age, particularly when orbital abnormalities or skeletal abnormalities are suspected. (See Sections 17.2.3, 17.3, and 17.7 for further details.)

REFERENCES

11. Hohler CW, Quetel TA: Comparison of ultrasound femur length and biparietal diameter in the late pregnancy. *Am J Obstet Gynecol* 1981;141:759.
12. Mayden KL, Tortora M, Berkowitz RL, et al: Orbital diameters: A new parameter for prenatal diagnosis and dating. *Am J Obstet Gynecol* 1982;144:298.
13. Jeanty P: Estimation of fetal age by long bone measurements. *J Ultrasound Med* 1983;1(suppl):189.

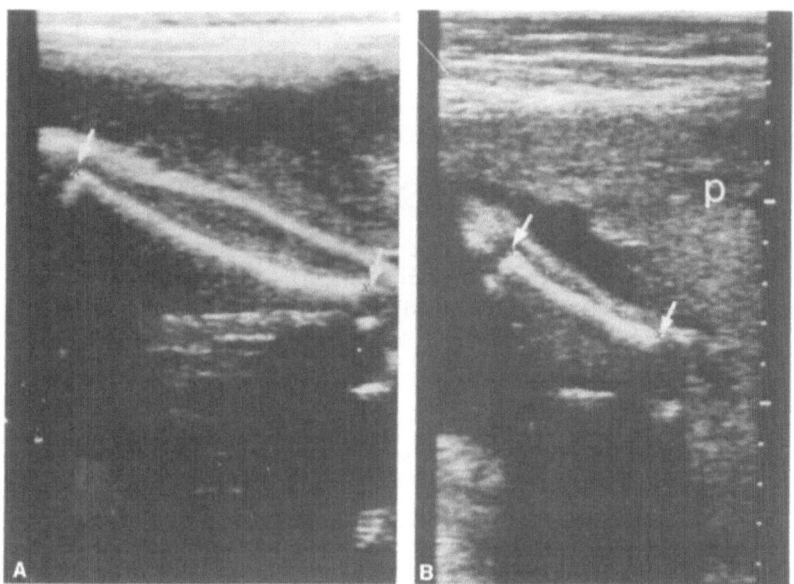

FIG. 7.2.5. MEASUREMENTS OF FEMORAL AND HUMERAL LENGTH

Longitudinal scan of the fetal femur (A) and humerus (B) indicating the point of measurement (X) for gestational dating. Placenta (p).

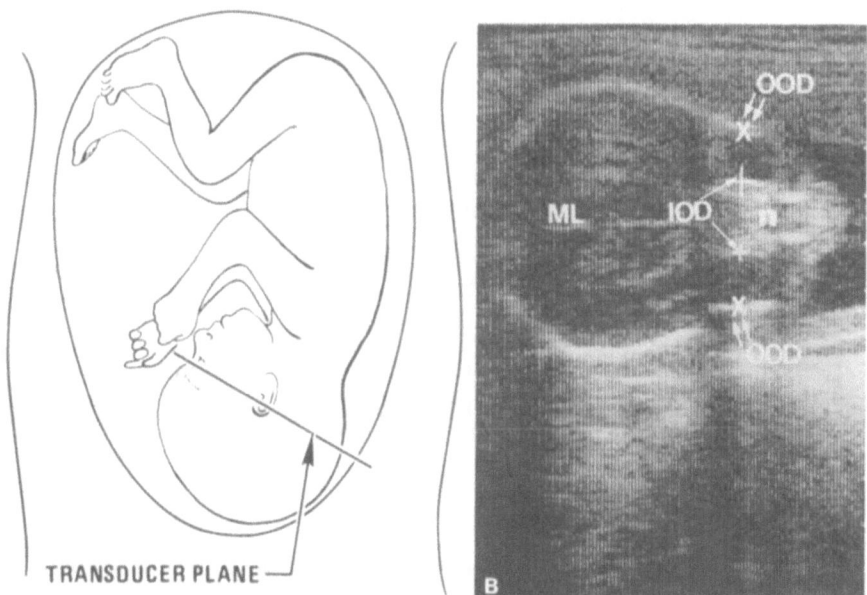

FIG. 7.2.6. ORBITAL MEASUREMENTS FOR ASSESSMENT OF GESTATIONAL AGE

(A) Schematic demonstrating the transducer plane for demonstrating orbital distance when the fetus is in occipital transverse head position. Coronal measurements of the orbits are also reliable indicators of gestational age.

(B) Oribtal measurements with the fetus in an occipital transverse position. Outer orbital distance (OOD), inner orbital distance (IOD), midline (ML), nasal bones (n).

From Mayden *et al.*[12]

7.3. THIRD TRIMESTER DATING

- During the third trimester of pregnancy, measurements of fetal BPD become less accurate because of the diminished growth rate of the fetal head and variations in fetal head position and shape. These variations in position and shape are related to molding and technical difficulties encountered with breech presentation and transverse lie.

- As a consequence of these and other factors, the single-measurement accuracy of the BPD decreases after 30 weeks to ± 3–3.5 weeks. Similarly, the femur length error after 30 weeks becomes equally long.[14]

- For these reasons it has been recommended that multiple parameters be used to assess fetal gestational age during the third trimester.[15] Other investigators disagree with inclusion of abdominal circumference for dating because of the possibility that fetal growth abnormalities may give false results.

- For 30–36 weeks, the following parameters are averaged[15]:

  o BPD
  o Abdominal circumference (see Fig. 7.3.1)
  o Femur length

- For 36 weeks to term, the following parameters are averaged[17]:

  o Head circumference
  o Abdominal circumference
  o Femur length

  Gestational assessment in the third trimester is therefore based on a number of fetal growth parameters (see Table 7.3.1).

- The *cephalic index* (CI) is used to establish the degree of molding of the fetal head, which allows the sonographer to determine whether the BPD should also be used for dating (see Table 7.3.2).

$$\text{Cephalic index (CI)} = \frac{\text{Biparietal diameter(BPD)}}{\text{Occipital frontal diameter (OFD)}} \times 100$$

  BPD is not to be used when the CI is either less than 75% or more than 85% (brachycephaly).[14]

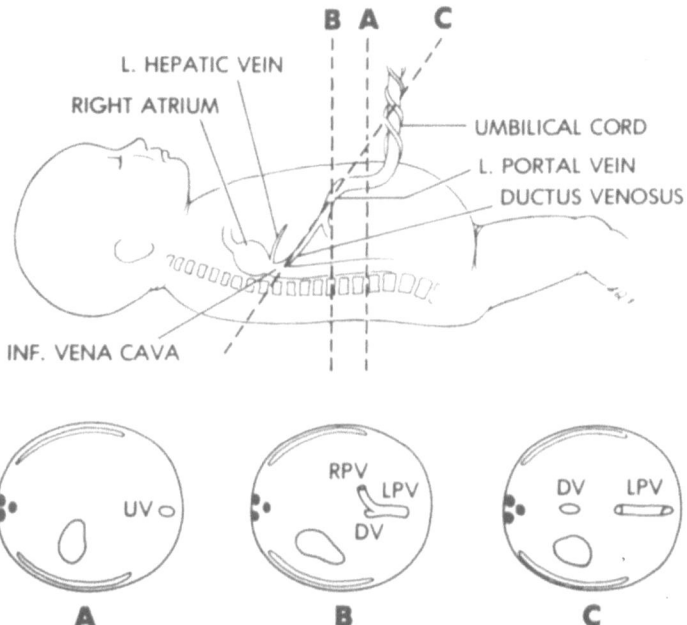

FIG. 7.3.1. HOW TO OBTAIN ABDOMINAL CIRCUMFERENCE

Diagrammatic representation of the umbilical venous blood supply to the fetus. The approximate plane of section for measurement of the abdominal diameter or circumference may be chosen on the basis of the appearance of the umbilical blood supply to the fetus.

(A) The scan is made at too low a level, as the umbilical vein (UV) sectioned along its short axis is adjacent to the anterior abdominal wall.

(B) This is the appropriate plane, demonstrating a short tubular segment of the umbilical segment of the left portal vein approximately one-third of the way posterior from the anterior abdominal wall. DV, ductus venosus.

(C) The plane is angulated, so that a long segment of the umbilical segment of the left portal vein (LPV) is seen.

From Deter *et al.*[16]

TABLE 7.3.1

Predicted Fetal Measurements at Specific Menstrual Weeks[a]

Menstrual age (weeks)	BPD (cm)	Head circumference (cm)	Abdominal circumference (cm)	Femur length (cm)
12	2.0	7.1	5.6	0.8
13	2.3	8.4	6.9	1.1
14	2.7	9.8	8.1	1.5
15	3.0	11.1	9.3	1.8
16	3.3	12.4	10.5	2.1
17	3.7	13.7	11.7	2.4
18	4.0	15.0	12.9	2.7
19	4.3	16.3	14.1	3.0
20	4.6	17.5	15.2	3.3
21	5.0	18.7	16.4	3.6
22	5.3	19.9	17.5	3.9
23	5.6	21.0	18.6	4.2
24	5.8	22.1	19.7	4.4
25	6.1	23.2	20.8	4.7
26	6.4	24.2	21.9	4.9
27	6.7	25.2	22.9	5.2
28	7.0	26.2	24.0	5.4
29	7.2	27.1	25.0	5.6
30	7.5	28.0	26.0	5.8
31	7.7	28.9	27.0	6.1
32	7.9	29.7	28.0	6.3
33	8.2	30.4	29.0	6.5
34	8.4	31.2	30.0	6.6
35	8.6	31.8	30.9	6.8
36	8.8	32.5	31.8	7.0
37	9.0	33.1	32.7	7.2
38	9.1	33.6	33.6	7.3
39	9.3	34.1	34.5	7.5
40	9.5	34.5	35.4	7.6

[a]From Hadlock et al.[17]

TABLE 7.3.2.
Predicted Biparietal Diameter and Weeks Gestation From the Inner and Outer Orbital Diameters[a]

BPD (cm)	Weeks gestation	IOD (cm)	OOD (cm)	BPD (cm)	Weeks gestation	IOD (cm)	OOD (cm)
1.9	11.6	0.5	1.3	5.8	24.3	1.6	4.1
2.0	11.6	0.5	1.4	5.9	24.3	1.6	4.2
2.1	12.1	0.6	1.5	6.0	24.7	1.6	4.3
2.2	12.6	0.6	1.6	6.1	25.2	1.6	4.3
2.3	12.6	0.6	1.7	6.2	25.2	1.6	4.4
2.4	13.1	0.7	1.7	6.3	25.7	1.7	4.4
2.5	13.6	0.7	1.8	6.4	26.2	1.7	4.5
2.6	13.6	0.7	1.9	6.5	26.2	1.7	4.5
2.7	14.1	0.8	2.0	6.6	26.7	1.7	4.6
2.8	14.6	0.8	2.1	6.7	27.2	1.7	4.6
2.9	14.6	0.8	2.1	6.8	27.6	1.7	4.7
3.0	15.0	0.9	2.2	6.9	28.1	1.7	4.7
3.1	15.5	0.9	2.3	7.0	28.6	1.8	4.8
3.2	15.5	0.9	2.4	7.1	29.1	1.8	4.8
3.3	16.0	1.0	2.5	7.3	29.6	1.8	4.9
3.4	16.5	1.0	2.5	7.4	30.0	1.8	5.0
3.5	16.5	1.0	2.6	7.5	30.6	1.8	5.0
3.6	17.0	1.0	2.7	7.6	31.0	1.8	5.1
3.7	17.5	1.1	2.7	7.7	31.5	1.8	5.1
3.8	17.9	1.1	2.8	7.8	32.0	1.8	5.2
4.0	18.4	1.2	3.0	7.9	32.5	1.9	5.2
4.2	18.9	1.2	3.1	8.0	33.0	1.9	5.3
4.3	19.4	1.2	3.2	8.2	33.5	1.9	5.4
4.4	19.4	1.3	3.2	8.3	34.0	1.9	5.4
4.5	19.9	1.3	3.3	8.4	34.4	1.9	5.4
4.6	20.4	1.3	3.4	8.5	35.0	1.9	5.5
4.7	20.4	1.3	3.4	8.6	35.4	1.9	5.5
4.8	20.9	1.4	3.5	8.8	35.9	1.9	5.6
4.9	21.3	1.4	3.6	8.9	36.4	1.9	5.6
5.0	21.3	1.4	3.6	9.0	36.9	1.9	5.7
5.1	21.8	1.4	3.7	9.1	37.3	1.9	5.7
5.2	22.3	1.4	3.8	9.2	37.8	1.9	5.8
5.3	22.3	1.5	3.8	9.3	38.3	1.9	5.8
5.4	22.8	1.5	3.9	9.4	38.8	1.9	5.8
5.5	23.3	1.5	4.0	9.6	39.3	1.9	5.9
5.6	23.3	1.5	4.0	9.7	39.8	1.9	5.9
5.7	23.8	1.5	4.1	—	—	—	—

[a] Biparietal diameter (BPD), inner orbital diameter (IOD), outer orbital diameter (OOD).
From Mayden *et al.*[12]

7.3.1. Abdominal Circumference

- Parameters for an adequate abdominal circumference (AC) are as follows:

  o The AC should be symmetrically circular.

  o It should be obtained just below the diaphragm at the bifurcation of the main portal vein into right and left portal vein[18] (see Section 4.7).

  o The level of the AC should include the fetal liver, spine, stomach, and umbilical portion of the portal system at the bifurcation (see Figs. 7.3.1–7.3.4 and Table 8.2.1).

  o Tables for AC refer to perimeter measurements used with a map reader (see Fig. 7.3.2).

- AC may at times be difficult to obtain or may be unreliable for any of several reasons:

  o Compression of the fetal abdomen due to oligohydramnios, malposition, fetal movements, congenital abnormalities

  o Spine-up, spine-down position of the fetus (see Figs. 7.3.4 and 7.3.5)

  o Nonvisualization of the fetal stomach (see Section 4.7)

  o Fetal ascites (see Chapters 10 and 11)

- AC is widely used in fetal weight estimation, as discussed in Section 8.2.

- AC will be the first parameter to be affected by IUGR or fetal macrosomia, as discussed in Sections 8.3.1 and 8.3.2.

- Previous terminology concerning the venous portal system of the fetus has recently been revised.[19] The above-listed parameters reflect this new terminology.

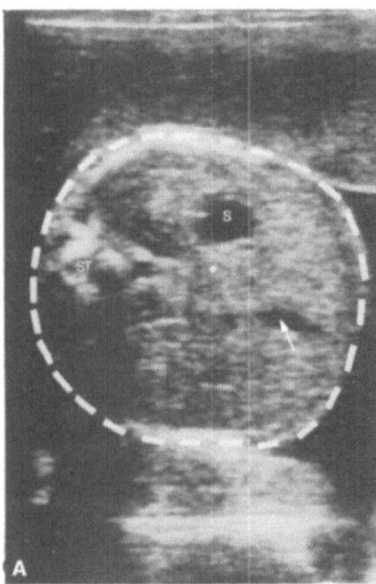 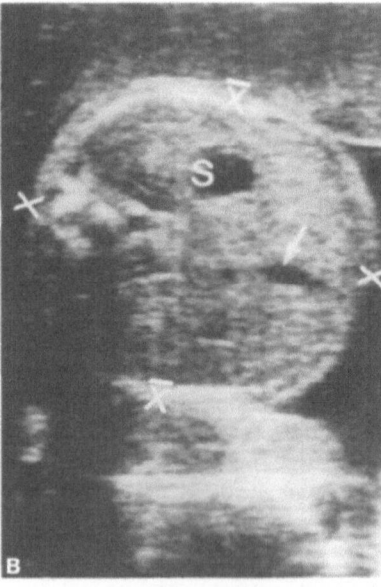

FIG. 7.3.2. CALCULATION OF ABDOMINAL CIRCUMFERENCE (AC)

Transverse scans (A,B) of the fetal abdomen at the level of the abdominal circumference. stomach (S), spine (ST), left portal vein (arrow).

AC can be measured by two methods:

(A) *Map reader*: AC (dotted lines) is calibrated into map units and multiplied by 10.

(B) *Formula*:
AC = anterior-posterior (AP) diameter (X) + transverse diameter (X̄) × 1.57

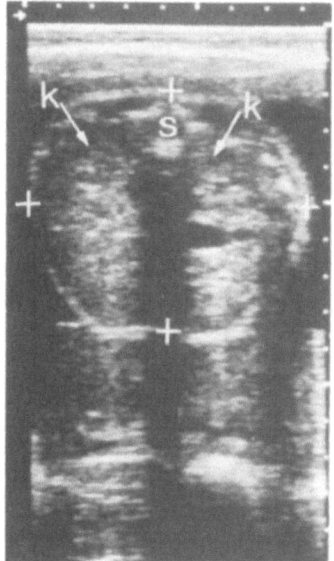

FIG. 7.3.3. ABDOMINAL CIRCUMFERENCE

Transverse scan through the fetal abdomen at the level of the abdominal circumference with the fetus in a spine-up (s) position. The upper poles of the fetal kidneys (k) are used as landmarks.

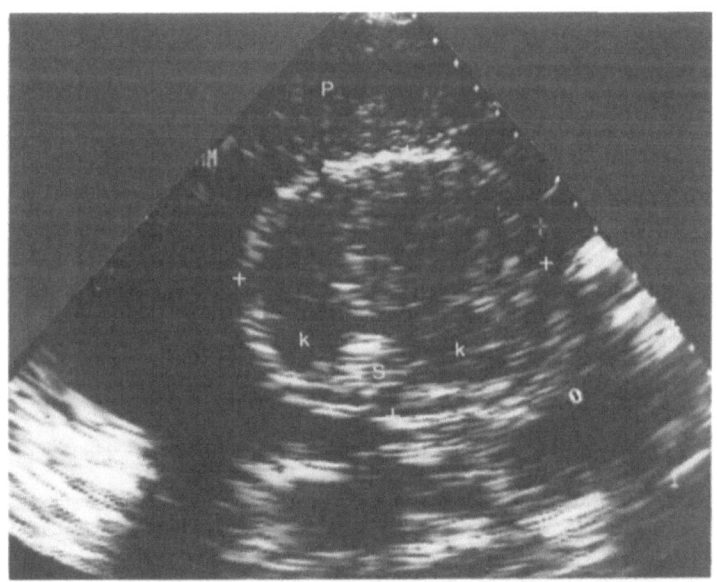

FIG. 7.3.4. ABDOMINAL CIRCUMFERENCE

Transverse scan through the fetal abdomen at the level of the abdominal circumference with the fetus in a spine-down (S) position. The upper poles of the fetal kidneys (k) are used as landmarks.

7.3.2. Head Circumference

- Parameters for an adequate head circumference (HC) are represented by a transverse scan through the fetal head at the appropriate level of a BPD. (For details, see Section 7.2.1 and Fig. 7.3.5.)

- HC represents a more reliable parameter of gestational age than BPD during late gestation because it is not affected by molding of the fetal head.

- In addition, HC is a most valuable parameter for the diagnosis of symmetric IUGR (see Section 8.3.1) as well as microcephaly.

7.3.3. Biparietal Diameter

The biparietal diameter (BPD), when employed during the third trimester, is obtained as described in Section 7.2.1.

7.3.4. Femur Length

Femur length, when used during the third trimester, is obtained as described in Section 7.2.2.

For summary scheme of pregnancy dating, see Fig. 7.3.6.

REFERENCES

14. Chervenak FA, Jeanty P, Hobbins JC: Current status of fetal age and growth assessment. *Clin Obstet Gynecol* 1983;10:423.
15. Hadlock FP, Deter RL, Harrist RB, et al: The use of ultrasound to determine fetal age—A review. *Med Ultrasound* 1983;7:95.
16. Deter RL, Hadlock FP, Harrist RB: Exaluation of normal fetal growth and the detection of intrauterine growth retardation, in Callen PW (ed): *Ultrasonography in Obstetrics and Gynecology*. Philadelphia, WB Saunders, 1983.
17. Hadlock FP, Deter RL, Harrist RB, et al: Computer assisted analysis of fetal age in the third trimester using multiple fetal growth parameters. *J. Clin Ultrasound* 1983;11:313.
18. Jeanty P, Romero R: *Obstetrical Ultrasound*. New York, McGraw-Hill, 1983.
19. Chinn, DH, Filly RA, Callen PW: Ultrasonic evaluation of fetal umbilical and hepatic vascular anatomy. *Radiology* 1982;144:153.

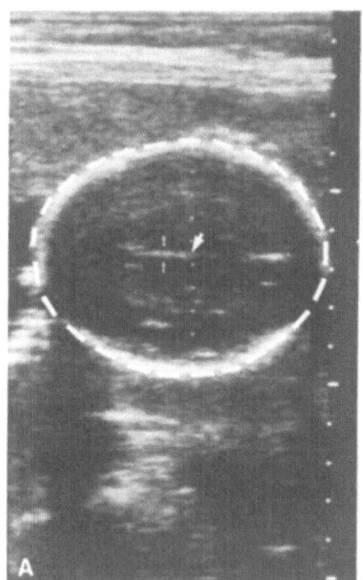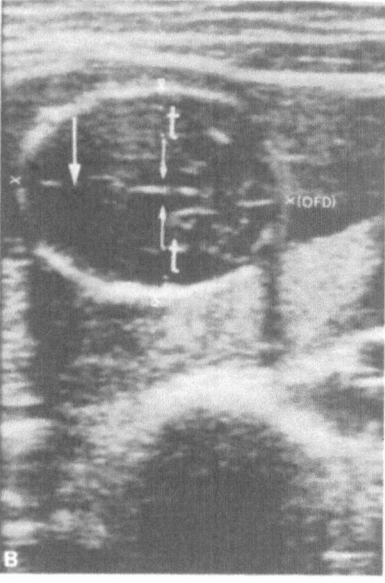

FIG. 7.3.5. CALCULATION OF HEAD CIRCUMFERENCE (HC) AND CEPHALIC INDEX

Transverse scans (A,B) through the fetal head at the level of the biparietal diameter for head circumference (HC) and cephalic index (CI). Thalami (t), midline (arrow). HC can be measured by two methods:

(A) *Map reader*: See Section 7.3.3.

(B) *Formula*:

HC = AP diameter (X) + (occipito-frontal diameter, OFD) + transverse diameter ($\bar{X}$) × 1.62

FIG. 7.3.6. SUMMARY SCHEME FOR PREGNANCY DATING BY SIMPLE SONOGRAPHIC EVALUATION

4–7 weeks	Gestational sac
6–13 weeks	Crown–rump length (CRL)
12–30 weeks	Biparietal diameter (BPD) Femur length (FL)
30–36 weeks	Biparietal diameter (BPD) Abdominal circumference (AC)* Femur length (FL)
36 weeks to term	Head circumference (HC) Abdominal circumference (AC)* Femur length (FL)

*According to Hadlock *et al.*[17] but disputed by others (see Section 7.3).

Chapter 8
Fetal Growth and Weight Estimation

8.1. NORMAL FETAL GROWTH

- The cost–benefit ratio for routine sonography for all pregnancies has remained controversial. While some European groups recommend cost efficiency in performing a routine baseline sonogram during the early mid-trimester in all patients, such an approach has not been accepted in the United States, as indicated by a recent National Institutes of Health Consensus Development Conference (1984).

- General consensus exists that an early baseline sonogram should be obtained in all pregnancies in which either clinical dating by other parameters seems unreliable or growth difficulties of the fetus(es) may be anticipated during the later course of pregnancy.

8.1.1. Methods for Evaluating Fetal Growth

Standard methods for gestational dating as outlined in Chapter 7 are also used for prospective estimation of fetal growth. These include different parameters, again depending on gestational age. (See the summarizing scheme for pregnancy dating in Fig. 7.3.7; see also Figs. 8.1.1 and 8.1.2.)

8.1.2. Timing of Sonography

- Excluding the practice of routine sonography during the early second trimester, certain principles may be applied to the process of dating patients in whom fetal growth difficulties are either noted clinically or are anticipated. Included among these principles are the following:

  1. If date of last menstrual period (LMP) is unknown or inaccurate, an initial sonogram is recommended as early as possible because of increased likelihood of dating error with advancing gestational age.

  2. The same principle applies if a date–size discrepancy of more than 2 weeks is noted.

  3. Similarly, an early baseline sonogram should be obtained whenever prospective growth difficulties of the fetus(es) may be expected. Such conditions are listed in Fig. 8.1.3.

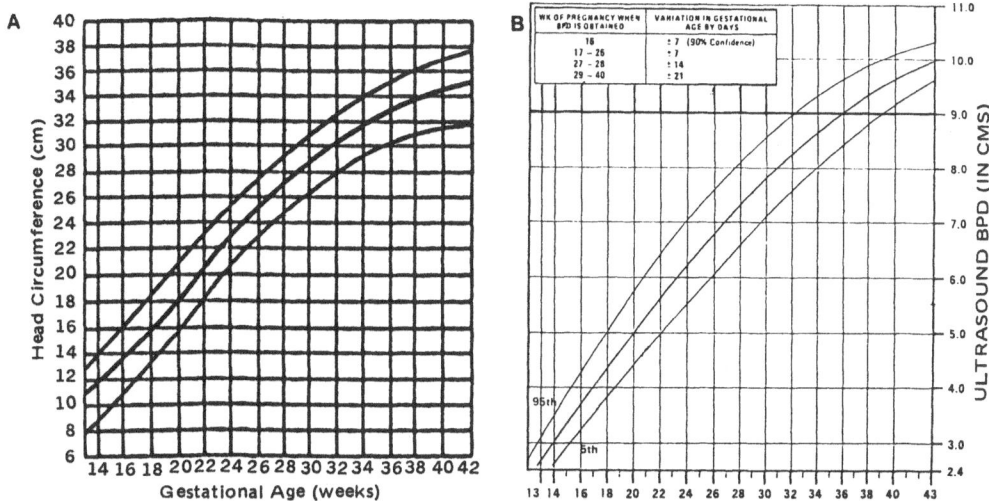

FIG. 8.1.1. FETAL GROWTH CURVES ACCORDING TO BIPARIETAL DIAMETER AND HEAD CIRCUMFERENCE

(A) Head circumference (HC) graph showing the expected growth pattern for the fetal head in the 5th, 50th, and 95th percentiles. From Metrewel.[3]

(B) Biparietal diameter (BPD) graph showing the expected growth pattern for the fetal head in the 5th, 50th, and 95th percentiles. From Sabbagha and Hughey.[2]

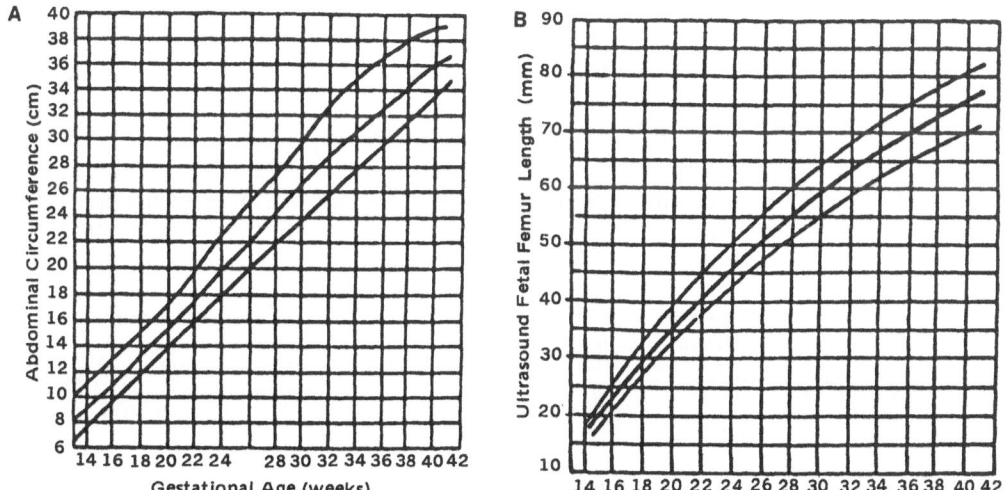

FIG. 8.1.2. FETAL GROWTH CURVES ACCORDING TO ABDOMINAL CIRCUMFERENCE[2] AND FEMUR LENGTH[3]

(A) Abdominal circumference (AC) graph showing the expected growth pattern for the fetal abdomen in 5th, 50th, and 95th percentiles.
From Metrewel.[3]

(B) Femur length (FL) graph showing the expected growth pattern for the fetal femur in the 5th, 50th, and 95th percentiles. From O'Brien and Queenan.[4]

CHAPTER 8 • FETAL GROWTH AND WEIGHT ESTIMATION

- After a baseline sonogram has been obtained, the timing of subsequent serial scans needs to be determined. The interval to the second sonogram will depend on the timing and outcome of the initial scan. Certain recommendations can be made but may vary from center to center (see Fig. 8.1.4):

1. Patient presenting with unknown dates late during the first trimester or early in second trimester (sonographically 10–20 weeks): Reschedule for growth reevaluation at 27–31 weeks. If no confounding problems surface in the patient and if her growth pattern appears normal, no further sonographic evaluation will be necessary.

2. Patient presenting with questionable dates at 10–20 weeks: If baseline sonogram confirms previously questionable LMP, no further sonographic evaluation will be necessary as long as no additional confounding factors arise.

3. Patient presenting with unknown or questionable dates at 21–30 weeks: The principle of the second scan remains the same as outlined under 1 and 2 above. However, the second scan has to be obtained sooner, depending on the originally determined gestational age.

    Example:
    First scan: 21 weeks   Follow-up: 28–30 weeks
               25 weeks   28–30 weeks
               29 weeks   31–33 weeks

    The interval between original and follow-up scan will decrease with increasing gestational age at first scan.
    o The BPD growth curve is the steepest before gestational weeks 27–28.
    o Thereafter, diverging growth between BPD and AC will become obvious, permitting the diagnosis of asymetric IUGR (see Section 8.3.1).
    Because of these factors, it seems beneficial to schedule follow-up scans in late-presenting patients before 30 weeks whenever possible.

4. A patient presenting for the first time after 31 weeks with unknown or questionable dates is recommended to undergo a follow-up scan at 2–4 weeks.

FIG. 8.1.3. INDICATIONS FOR EARLY BASELINE SONOGRAPHY WITH EXPECTED GROWTH AND/OR DATING DIFFICULTIES

Morbid maternal obesity

Erythroblastosis fetalis (Rh disease)

Necessity for timed delivery

  Previous cesarean section
  Previous uterine surgery
  Abnormal presentation

X-ray exposure

Medications

  · Coumadin
  Dilantin
  Trimethadione
  Aminopterin

High altitude

Multiple gestation (see Chapter 12)

Previous growth-retarded child

Maternal smoking

Maternal substance abuse (including alcohol)

Maternal medical diseases

  Chronic hypertension
  Diabetes mellitus
  Renal diseases
  Systemic lupus erythematosus
  Severe anemias
  Severe cardiac diseases
  Malabsorption
  Severe asthma
  Chronic liver disease

FIG. 8.1.4. FLOW CHART FOR SONOGRAPHIC SCHEDULING OF PATIENTS WITH QUESTIONABLE OR UNKNOWN DATES

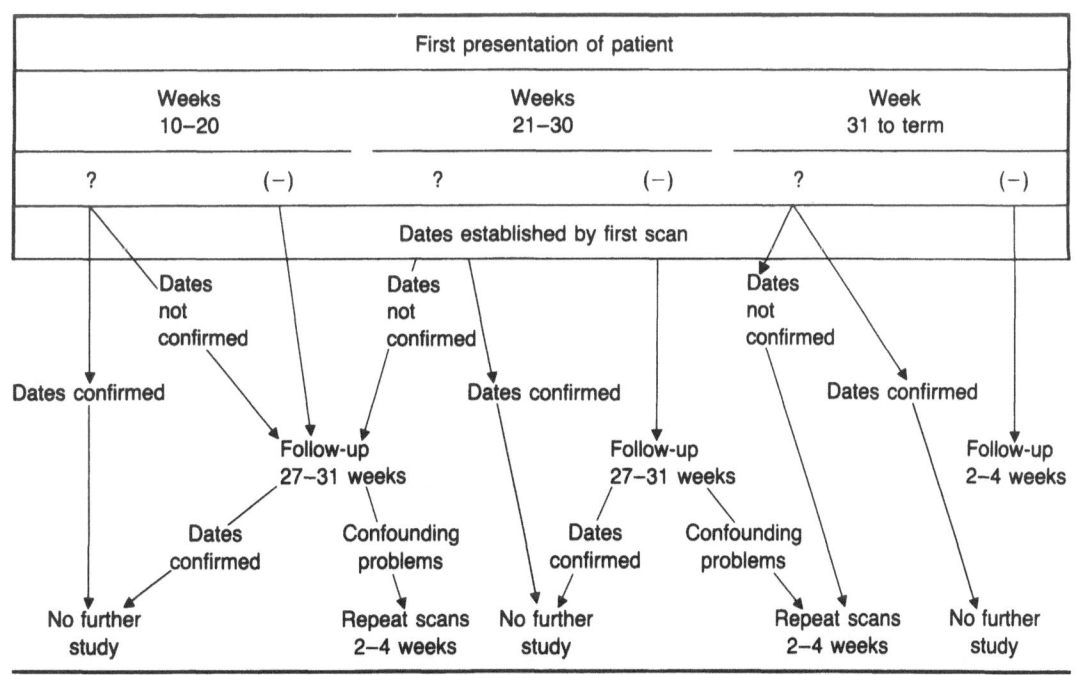

(?) Questionable dates; (−) unknown dates.

8.2. ESTIMATION OF FETAL WEIGHT

- Estimation of fetal weight (EFW) has become possible with acceptable accuracy.[1]

- The accuracy of the EFW decreases at the weight extremes, i.e., very-low-weight infants and severely macrosomic fetuses.

- The technique for evaluating EFW includes the acquisition of BPD, with a normal cephalic index (CI) (see Section 7.3) and abdominal circumference (AC). (For the measurement of and equations governing standard BPD and AC, see Sections 7.2 and 7.3.)

- Once BPD and AC are obtained, EFW can be predicted by cross-referencing from any of many available nomograms (see Table 8.2.1).

- The potential error in assessing EFW is equal to ±106 g/kg fetal body weight.[5]

REFERENCES

1. Shepard MJ, Richards VA, Berkowitz RL, et al: An evaluation of two equations for predicting fetal weight by ultrasound. *Am J Obstet Gynecol* 1982;142:47.
2. Sabbagha RE, Hughey M: Standardization of sonar cephalometry and gestational age. *Obstet Gynecol* 1978;52:402.
3. Metrewel C: *Practical Abdominal Ultrasound*. London, Heinemann, 1978.
4. O'Brien GD, Queenan JT: Ultrasound fetal femur length in relation to intrauterine growth retardation. *Am J Obstet Gynecol* 1982;144:35.
5. Warsof SL, Gohari P, Berkowitz RL, et al: The estimation of fetal weight by computer assisted analysis. *Am J Obstet Gynecol* 1977;128:881.

TABLE 8.2.1
Estimated Fetal Weights[a]

Biparietal diameters	Abdominal circumferences																
	15.5	16.0	16.5	17.0	17.5	18.0	18.5	19.0	19.5	20.0	20.5	21.0	21.5	22.0	22.5	23.0	23.5
3.1	224	234	244	255	267	279	291	304	318	332	346	362	378	395	412	431	450
3.2	231	241	251	263	274	286	299	312	326	340	355	371	388	405	423	441	461
3.3	237	248	259	270	282	294	307	321	335	349	365	381	397	415	433	452	472
3.4	244	255	266	278	290	302	316	329	344	359	374	391	408	425	444	463	483
3.5	251	262	274	285	298	311	324	338	353	368	384	401	418	436	455	475	495
3.6	259	270	281	294	306	319	333	347	362	378	394	411	429	447	466	486	507
3.7	266	278	290	302	315	328	342	357	372	388	404	422	440	458	478	498	519
3.8	274	286	298	310	324	337	352	366	382	398	415	432	451	470	490	510	532
3.9	282	294	306	319	333	347	361	376	392	409	426	444	462	482	502	523	545
4.0	290	303	315	328	342	356	371	386	403	419	437	455	474	494	514	536	558
4.1	299	311	324	338	352	366	381	397	413	430	448	467	486	506	527	549	572
4.2	308	320	333	347	361	376	392	408	424	442	460	479	498	519	540	562	585
4.3	317	330	343	357	371	387	402	419	436	453	472	491	511	532	554	576	600
4.4	326	339	353	367	382	397	413	430	447	465	484	504	524	545	567	590	614
4.5	335	349	363	377	393	408	425	442	459	478	497	517	538	559	581	605	629
4.6	345	359	373	388	404	420	436	454	472	490	510	530	551	573	596	620	644
4.7	355	369	384	399	415	431	448	466	484	503	523	544	565	588	611	635	660
4.8	366	380	395	410	426	443	460	478	497	517	537	558	580	602	626	650	676
4.9	379	391	406	422	438	455	473	491	510	530	551	572	594	617	641	666	692
5.0	387	402	418	434	451	468	486	505	524	544	565	587	610	633	657	683	709
5.1	399	414	430	446	463	481	499	518	538	559	580	602	625	649	674	699	726
5.2	410	426	442	459	476	494	513	532	552	573	595	618	641	665	690	717	744
5.3	422	438	455	472	489	508	527	547	567	589	611	634	657	682	708	734	762
5.4	435	451	468	485	503	522	541	561	582	604	627	650	674	699	725	752	780
5.5	447	464	481	499	517	536	556	577	598	620	643	667	691	717	743	771	799
5.6	461	477	495	513	532	551	571	592	614	636	660	684	709	735	762	789	818
5.7	474	491	509	527	547	566	587	608	630	653	677	701	727	753	780	809	838
5.8	488	505	524	542	562	582	603	625	647	670	695	719	745	772	800	829	858
5.9	502	520	539	558	578	598	619	642	664	688	713	738	764	792	820	849	879
6.0	517	535	554	573	594	615	636	659	682	706	731	757	784	811	840	870	900
6.1	532	550	570	590	610	632	654	677	700	725	750	777	804	832	861	891	922
6.2	547	566	586	606	627	649	672	695	719	744	770	797	824	853	882	913	945
6.3	563	583	603	624	645	667	690	714	738	764	790	817	845	874	904	935	967
6.4	580	600	620	641	663	686	709	733	758	784	811	838	867	896	927	958	991
6.5	597	617	638	659	682	705	728	753	778	805	832	860	889	919	950	982	1,015
6.6	614	635	656	678	701	724	748	773	799	826	853	882	911	942	973	1,006	1,039
6.7	632	653	675	697	720	744	769	794	820	848	876	905	935	965	997	1,030	1,065
6.8	651	672	694	717	740	765	790	816	842	870	898	928	958	990	1,022	1,056	1,090
6.9	670	691	714	737	761	786	811	838	865	893	922	952	983	1,015	1,048	1,082	1,117
7.0	689	711	734	758	782	807	833	860	888	916	946	976	1,008	1,040	1,074	1,108	1,144
7.1	709	732	755	779	804	830	856	883	912	941	971	1,002	1,033	1,066	1,100	1,135	1,171
7.2	730	763	777	801	827	853	880	907	936	965	996	1,027	1,060	1,093	1,128	1,163	1,200
7.3	751	775	799	824	850	876	904	932	961	991	1,022	1,054	1,087	1,121	1,156	1,192	1,229
7.4	773	797	822	847	874	901	928	957	987	1,017	1,049	1,081	1,114	1,149	1,184	1,221	1,259
7.5	796	820	845	871	898	925	954	983	1,013	1,044	1,076	1,109	1,143	1,178	1,214	1,251	1,289
7.6	819	844	870	896	923	951	980	1,009	1,040	1,072	1,104	1,137	1,172	1,207	1,244	1,281	1,320
7.7	843	868	894	921	949	977	1,007	1,037	1,068	1,100	1,133	1,167	1,202	1,238	1,275	1,313	1,352
7.8	868	894	920	947	975	1,004	1,034	1,065	1,096	1,129	1,162	1,197	1,232	1,269	1,306	1,345	1,385
7.9	893	919	946	974	1,003	1,032	1,062	1,094	1,126	1,159	1,193	1,228	1,264	1,301	1,339	1,378	1,418
8.0	919	946	973	1,002	1,031	1,061	1,091	1,123	1,156	1,189	1,224	1,259	1,296	1,333	1,372	1,412	1,453
8.1	946	973	1,001	1,030	1,060	1,090	1,121	1,153	1,187	1,221	1,256	1,292	1,329	1,367	1,406	1,446	1,488
8.2	974	1,001	1,030	1,059	1,089	1,120	1,152	1,185	1,218	1,253	1,288	1,325	1,363	1,401	1,441	1,482	1,524
8.3	1,002	1,030	1,059	1,089	1,120	1,151	1,183	1,217	1,251	1,286	1,322	1,359	1,397	1,436	1,477	1,518	1,561
8.4	1,032	1,060	1,090	1,120	1,151	1,183	1,216	1,249	1,284	1,320	1,356	1,394	1,433	1,473	1,513	1,555	1,599
8.5	1,062	1,091	1,121	1,151	1,183	1,216	1,249	1,283	1,318	1,355	1,392	1,430	1,469	1,510	1,551	1,594	1,637
8.6	1,093	1,122	1,153	1,184	1,216	1,249	1,283	1,318	1,354	1,390	1,428	1,467	1,507	1,548	1,589	1,633	1,677
8.7	1,125	1,155	1,186	1,218	1,250	1,284	1,318	1,353	1,390	1,427	1,465	1,505	1,545	1,586	1,629	1,673	1,717
8.8	1,157	1,188	1,220	1,252	1,285	1,319	1,354	1,390	1,427	1,465	1,504	1,543	1,584	1,626	1,669	1,714	1,759
8.9	1,191	1,222	1,254	1,287	1,321	1,356	1,391	1,428	1,465	1,503	1,543	1,583	1,625	1,667	1,711	1,756	1,802
9.0	1,226	1,258	1,290	1,324	1,358	1,393	1,429	1,456	1,504	1,543	1,583	1,624	1,666	1,709	1,753	1,799	1,845
9.1	1,262	1,294	1,327	1,361	1,396	1,432	1,468	1,506	1,544	1,584	1,624	1,666	1,708	1,752	1,797	1,843	1,890
9.2	1,299	1,332	1,365	1,400	1,435	1,471	1,508	1,546	1,586	1,626	1,667	1,709	1,752	1,796	1,841	1,888	1,936
9.3	1,337	1,370	1,404	1,439	1,475	1,512	1,550	1,588	1,628	1,668	1,710	1,753	1,796	1,841	1,887	1,934	1,982
9.4	1,376	1,410	1,444	1,480	1,516	1,554	1,592	1,631	1,671	1,712	1,755	1,798	1,842	1,887	1,934	1,982	2,030
9.5	1,416	1,450	1,486	1,522	1,559	1,597	1,635	1,675	1,716	1,758	1,800	1,844	1,889	1,935	1,982	2,030	2,080
9.6	1,457	1,492	1,528	1,565	1,602	1,641	1,680	1,720	1,762	1,804	1,847	1,892	1,937	1,984	2,031	2,080	2,130
9.7	1,500	1,535	1,572	1,609	1,547	1,686	1,726	1,767	1,809	1,852	1,895	1,940	1,986	2,033	2,082	2,131	2,181
9.8	1,544	1,580	1,617	1,654	1,693	1,733	1,773	1,815	1,857	1,900	1,945	1,990	2,037	2,085	2,133	2,183	2,234
9.9	1,589	1,625	1,663	1,701	1,740	1,781	1,822	1,864	1,907	1,951	1,996	2,042	2,086	2,137	2,186	2,237	2,288
10.0	1,635	1,672	1,710	1,749	1,789	1,830	1,871	1,914	1,958	2,002	2,048	2,094	2,142	2,191	2,241	2,292	2,344

[a]Log (birth weight) = $-1.7942 + 0.166$ (BPD) $+ 0.032$ (AC) $- 2.646$ (BPD × AC/1000.
SD = 106.0 g/kg of body weight. From Shepard et al.[1]

TABLE 8.2.1. (Continued)

Biparietal diameters	Abdominal circumferences																
	24.0	24.5	25.0	25.5	26.0	26.5	27.0	27.5	28.0	28.5	29.0	29.5	30.0	30.5	31.0	31.5	32.0
3.1	470	491	513	536	559	584	610	638	666	696	726	759	793	828	865	903	943
3.2	481	502	525	548	572	597	624	651	680	710	742	774	809	844	882	921	961
3.3	493	514	537	560	585	611	638	666	695	725	757	790	825	861	899	938	979
3.4	504	526	549	573	598	624	652	680	710	740	773	806	841	878	916	956	998
3.5	517	539	562	587	612	638	666	695	725	756	789	823	858	896	934	975	1,017
3.6	529	552	575	600	626	653	681	710	740	772	805	840	876	913	953	993	1,036
3.7	542	565	589	614	640	667	696	725	756	788	822	857	893	931	971	1,012	1,056
3.8	554	578	602	628	654	682	711	741	772	805	839	874	911	950	990	1,032	1,076
3.9	568	592	616	642	669	697	727	757	789	822	856	892	930	969	1,009	1,052	1,096
4.0	581	606	631	657	684	713	743	773	806	839	874	911	949	988	1,029	1,072	1,117
4.1	595	620	645	672	700	729	759	790	828	857	892	929	968	1,008	1,049	1,093	1,138
4.2	609	634	660	688	716	745	776	807	841	875	911	948	987	1,028	1,070	1,114	1,159
4.3	624	649	676	703	732	762	793	825	859	893	930	968	1,007	1,048	1,091	1,135	1,181
4.4	639	665	692	719	749	779	810	843	877	912	949	987	1,027	1,069	1,112	1,157	1,204
4.5	654	680	708	736	765	796	828	861	896	932	969	1,008	1,048	1,090	1,134	1,179	1,226
4.6	670	696	724	753	783	814	846	880	915	951	989	1,028	1,069	1,112	1,156	1,202	1,249
4.7	686	713	741	770	801	832	865	899	934	971	1,010	1,049	1,091	1,134	1,178	1,225	1,273
4.8	702	730	758	788	819	851	884	919	954	992	1,031	1,071	1,113	1,156	1,201	1,248	1,297
4.9	719	747	776	806	837	870	903	938	975	1,013	1,052	1,093	1,135	1,179	1,225	1,272	1,322
5.0	736	765	794	824	856	889	923	959	996	1,034	1,074	1,115	1,158	1,203	1,249	1,297	1,347
5.1	754	783	812	843	876	909	944	980	1,017	1,056	1,096	1,138	1,181	1,226	1,273	1,322	1,372
5.2	772	801	831	863	895	929	964	1,001	1,039	1,078	1,119	1,161	1,205	1,251	1,298	1,347	1,398
5.3	790	820	851	883	916	950	986	1,023	1,061	1,101	1,142	1,185	1,229	1,276	1,323	1,373	1,425
5.4	809	839	870	903	936	971	1,007	1,045	1,084	1,124	1,166	1,209	1,254	1,301	1,349	1,399	1,452
5.5	828	859	891	924	958	993	1,030	1,068	1,107	1,148	1,190	1,234	1,279	1,327	1,376	1,426	1,479
5.6	848	879	911	945	979	1,015	1,052	1,091	1,131	1,172	1,215	1,259	1,305	1,353	1,402	1,454	1,507
5.7	869	900	933	966	1,001	1,038	1,075	1,114	1,155	1,197	1,240	1,285	1,332	1,380	1,430	1,482	1,535
5.8	889	921	954	989	1,024	1,061	1,099	1,139	1,180	1,222	1,266	1,311	1,358	1,407	1,458	1,510	1,564
5.9	911	943	977	1,011	1,047	1,085	1,123	1,163	1,205	1,248	1,292	1,338	1,386	1,435	1,486	1,539	1,594
6.0	932	965	999	1,035	1,071	1,109	1,148	1,189	1,231	1,274	1,319	1,366	1,414	1,464	1,515	1,569	1,624
6.1	955	988	1,023	1,058	1,095	1,134	1,173	1,214	1,257	1,301	1,346	1,393	1,442	1,493	1,545	1,599	1,655
6.2	977	1,011	1,046	1,083	1,120	1,159	1,199	1,241	1,284	1,328	1,374	1,422	1,471	1,522	1,575	1,630	1,686
6.3	1,001	1,035	1,071	1,107	1,145	1,185	1,226	1,268	1,311	1,356	1,403	1,451	1,501	1,552	1,606	1,661	1,718
6.4	1,025	1,059	1,096	1,133	1,171	1,211	1,253	1,295	1,339	1,385	1,432	1,481	1,531	1,583	1,637	1,693	1,751
6.5	1,049	1,084	1,121	1,159	1,198	1,238	1,280	1,323	1,368	1,414	1,462	1,511	1,562	1,615	1,669	1,725	1,784
6.6	1,074	1,110	1,147	1,185	1,225	1,266	1,308	1,352	1,397	1,444	1,492	1,542	1,594	1,647	1,702	1,759	1,817
6.7	1,100	1,136	1,174	1,213	1,253	1,294	1,337	1,381	1,427	1,474	1,523	1,574	1,626	1,679	1,735	1,792	1,852
6.8	1,126	1,163	1,201	1,241	1,281	1,323	1,367	1,411	1,458	1,505	1,555	1,606	1,658	1,713	1,769	1,827	1,887
6.9	1,153	1,190	1,229	1,269	1,310	1,353	1,397	1,442	1,489	1,537	1,587	1,639	1,692	1,747	1,803	1,862	1,922
7.0	1,181	1,219	1,258	1,298	1,340	1,383	1,427	1,473	1,521	1,570	1,620	1,672	1,726	1,781	1,839	1,898	1,959
7.1	1,209	1,247	1,287	1,328	1,370	1,414	1,459	1,505	1,553	1,603	1,654	1,706	1,761	1,817	1,875	1,934	1,996
7.2	1,238	1,277	1,317	1,358	1,401	1,445	1,491	1,538	1,586	1,636	1,688	1,741	1,796	1,853	1,911	1,971	2,044
7.3	1,267	1,307	1,348	1,390	1,433	1,478	1,524	1,571	1,620	1,671	1,723	1,777	1,832	1,890	1,948	2,009	2,072
7.4	1,297	1,338	1,379	1,421	1,465	1,511	1,557	1,605	1,655	1,706	1,759	1,813	1,869	1,927	1,987	2,048	2,111
7.5	1,328	1,369	1,411	1,454	1,499	1,544	1,592	1,640	1,690	1,742	1,795	1,850	1,907	1,965	2,025	2,087	2,151
7.6	1,360	1,401	1,444	1,487	1,533	1,579	1,627	1,676	1,727	1,779	1,833	1,888	1,945	2,004	2,065	2,127	2,192
7.7	1,393	1,434	1,477	1,522	1,567	1,614	1,663	1,712	1,764	1,816	1,871	1,927	1,985	2,044	2,105	2,168	2,233
7.8	1,426	1,468	1,512	1,557	1,603	1,650	1,699	1,749	1,801	1,855	1,910	1,966	2,025	2,085	2,146	2,210	2,275
7.9	1,460	1,503	1,547	1,592	1,639	1,687	1,737	1,787	1,840	1,894	1,949	2,006	2,065	2,126	2,188	2,252	2,318
8.0	1,495	1,538	1,583	1,629	1,676	1,725	1,775	1,826	1,879	1,934	1,990	2,048	2,107	2,168	2,231	2,296	2,362
8.1	1,531	1,575	1,620	1,666	1,714	1,763	1,814	1,866	1,919	1,975	2,031	2,089	2,149	2,211	2,275	2,340	2,407
8.2	1,567	1,612	1,657	1,704	1,753	1,803	1,854	1,906	1,960	2,016	2,073	2,132	2,193	2,255	2,319	2,385	2,462
8.3	1,605	1,650	1,696	1,744	1,793	1,843	1,895	1,948	2,002	2,059	2,116	2,176	2,237	2,300	2,364	2,431	2,499
8.4	1,643	1,689	1,735	1,784	1,833	1,884	1,936	1,990	2,045	2,102	2,160	2,220	2,282	2,345	2,410	2,477	2,546
8.5	1,682	1,728	1,776	1,825	1,875	1,926	1,979	2,033	2,089	2,146	2,205	2,266	2,328	2,392	2,457	2,525	2,594
8.6	1,722	1,769	1,817	1,866	1,917	1,969	2,022	2,077	2,134	2,192	2,251	2,312	2,375	2,439	2,505	2,573	2,643
8.7	1,764	1,811	1,859	1,909	1,960	2,013	2,067	2,122	2,179	2,238	2,298	2,359	2,423	2,488	2,554	2,623	2,693
8.8	1,806	1,854	1,903	1,953	2,005	2,058	2,113	2,169	2,226	2,285	2,346	2,408	2,472	2,537	2,604	2,673	2,744
8.9	1,849	1,897	1,947	1,998	2,050	2,104	2,159	2,216	2,274	2,333	2,394	2,457	2,521	2,587	2,655	2,725	2,796
9.0	1,893	1,942	1,992	2,044	2,097	2,151	2,207	2,264	2,322	2,382	2,444	2,507	2,572	2,639	2,707	2,777	2,849
9.1	1,938	1,988	2,039	2,091	2,144	2,199	2,255	2,313	2,372	2,433	2,495	2,559	2,624	2,691	2,760	2,830	2,903
9.2	1,984	2,035	2,086	2,139	2,193	2,248	2,305	2,363	2,423	2,484	2,547	2,611	2,677	2,744	2,814	2,885	2,958
9.3	2,032	2,083	2,135	2,188	2,242	2,298	2,356	2,414	2,475	2,536	2,599	2,664	2,731	2,799	2,869	2,940	3,014
9.4	2,080	2,132	2,184	2,238	2,293	2,350	2,407	2,467	2,527	2,590	2,653	2,719	2,786	2,854	2,925	2,997	3,070
9.5	2,130	2,182	2,235	2,289	2,345	2,402	2,460	2,520	2,582	2,644	2,709	2,774	2,842	2,911	2,982	3,054	3,129
9.6	2,181	2,233	2,287	2,342	2,398	2,456	2,515	2,575	2,637	2,700	2,765	2,831	2,899	2,969	3,040	3,113	3,188
9.7	2,233	2,286	2,340	2,396	2,452	2,510	2,570	2,631	2,693	2,757	2,822	2,889	2,958	3,028	3,099	3,173	3,248
9.8	2,286	2,340	2,395	2,451	2,508	2,567	2,627	2,688	2,751	2,815	2,881	2,948	3,017	3,088	3,160	3,234	3,309
9.9	2,341	2,395	2,450	2,507	2,565	2,624	2,684	2,746	2,810	2,874	2,941	3,009	3,078	3,149	3,222	3,296	3,372
10.0	2,397	2,452	2,507	2,564	2,623	2,682	2,743	2,806	2,870	2,935	3,002	3,070	3,140	3,211	3,285	3,359	3,436

TABLE 8.2.1. (*Continued*)

Biparietal diameters	Abdominal circumferences															
	32.5	33.0	33.5	34.0	34.5	35.0	35.5	36.0	36.5	37.0	37.5	38.0	38.5	39.0	39.5	40.0
3.1	985	1,029	1,075	1,123	1,173	1,225	1,279	1,336	1,396	1,458	1,523	1,591	1,661	1,735	1,812	1,893
3.2	1,004	1,048	1,094	1,143	1,193	1,246	1,301	1,358	1,418	1,481	1,546	1,615	1,686	1,761	1,838	1,920
3.3	1,022	1,067	1,114	1,163	1,214	1,267	1,323	1,381	1,441	1,504	1,570	1,639	1,711	1,786	1,865	1,946
3.4	1,041	1,087	1,134	1,183	1,235	1,289	1,345	1,403	1,464	1,528	1,595	1,664	1,737	1,812	1,891	1,973
3.5	1,061	1,107	1,154	1,204	1,256	1,311	1,367	1,426	1,488	1,552	1,619	1,689	1,762	1,839	1,918	2,001
3.6	1,080	1,127	1,175	1,226	1,278	1,333	1,390	1,450	1,512	1,577	1,645	1,715	1,789	1,865	1,945	2,029
3.7	1,101	1,147	1,196	1,247	1,300	1,356	1,413	1,474	1,536	1,602	1,670	1,741	1,815	1,893	1,973	2,057
3.8	1,121	1,168	1,218	1,269	1,323	1,379	1,437	1,498	1,561	1,627	1,696	1,768	1,842	1,920	2,001	2,086
3.9	1,142	1,190	1,240	1,292	1,346	1,402	1,461	1,523	1,586	1,653	1,722	1,794	1,870	1,948	2,030	2,115
4.0	1,163	1,212	1,262	1,315	1,369	1,426	1,486	1,548	1,612	1,679	1,749	1,822	1,898	1,977	2,059	2,145
4.1	1,185	1,234	1,285	1,338	1,393	1,451	1,511	1,573	1,638	1,706	1,776	1,849	1,926	2,005	2,088	2,174
4.2	1,207	1,256	1,308	1,361	1,417	1,475	1,536	1,599	1,664	1,733	1,804	1,878	1,954	2,035	2,118	2,205
4.3	1,229	1,279	1,331	1,385	1,442	1,500	1,562	1,625	1,691	1,760	1,832	1,906	1,984	2,064	2,148	2,236
4.4	1,252	1,303	1,355	1,410	1,467	1,526	1,588	1,652	1,718	1,788	1,860	1,935	2,013	2,094	2,179	2,267
4.5	1,275	1,326	1,380	1,435	1,492	1,552	1,614	1,679	1,746	1,816	1,889	1,964	2,043	2,125	2,210	2,298
4.6	1,299	1,351	1,404	1,460	1,518	1,579	1,641	1,706	1,774	1,845	1,918	1,994	2,073	2,156	2,241	2,330
4.7	1,323	1,375	1,430	1,486	1,545	1,605	1,669	1,734	1,803	1,874	1,948	2,024	2,104	2,187	2,273	2,363
4.8	1,348	1,401	1,455	1,512	1,571	1,633	1,697	1,763	1,832	1,904	1,978	2,055	2,136	2,219	2,306	2,396
4.9	1,373	1,426	1,482	1,539	1,599	1,661	1,725	1,792	1,861	1,934	2,009	2,086	2,167	2,251	2,339	2,429
5.0	1,399	1,452	1,508	1,566	1,626	1,689	1,754	1,821	1,891	1,964	2,040	2,118	2,200	2,284	2,372	2,463
5.1	1,425	1,479	1,535	1,594	1,655	1,718	1,783	1,851	1,922	1,995	2,071	2,150	2,232	2,317	2,406	2,498
5.2	1,451	1,506	1,563	1,622	1,683	1,747	1,813	1,882	1,953	2,027	2,103	2,183	2,266	2,351	2,440	2,532
5.3	1,478	1,533	1,591	1,651	1,713	1,777	1,843	1,913	1,984	2,059	2,136	2,216	2,299	2,386	2,475	2,568
5.4	1,506	1,562	1,620	1,680	1,742	1,807	1,874	1,944	2,016	2,091	2,169	2,250	2,333	2,420	2,510	2,604
5.5	1,534	1,590	1,649	1,710	1,773	1,838	1,906	1,976	2,049	2,124	2,203	2,284	2,368	2,456	2,546	2,640
5.6	1,562	1,619	1,678	1,740	1,803	1,869	1,938	2,008	2,082	2,158	2,237	2,319	2,403	2,491	2,582	2,677
5.7	1,591	1,649	1,709	1,770	1,835	1,901	1,970	2,041	2,115	2,192	2,272	2,354	2,439	2,528	2,619	2,714
5.8	1,621	1,679	1,739	1,802	1,866	1,934	2,003	2,075	2,150	2,227	2,307	2,390	2,475	2,564	2,657	2,752
5.9	1,651	1,710	1,770	1,834	1,899	1,966	2,037	2,109	2,184	2,262	2,342	2,426	2,512	2,602	2,694	2,790
6.0	1,682	1,741	1,802	1,866	1,932	2,000	2,071	2,144	2,219	2,298	2,379	2,463	2,550	2,640	2,733	2,829
6.1	1,713	1,773	1,835	1,899	1,965	2,034	2,105	2,179	2,255	2,334	2,416	2,500	2,588	2,678	2,772	2,869
6.2	1,745	1,805	1,868	1,932	1,999	2,069	2,140	2,215	2,291	2,371	2,453	2,538	2,626	2,717	2,811	2,909
6.3	1,777	1,838	1,901	1,967	2,034	2,104	2,176	2,251	2,328	2,408	2,491	2,577	2,665	2,757	2,851	2,949
6.4	1,810	1,872	1,935	2,001	2,069	2,140	2,213	2,288	2,366	2,446	2,530	2,616	2,705	2,797	2,892	2,991
6.5	1,844	1,906	1,970	2,037	2,105	2,176	2,250	2,326	2,404	2,485	2,569	2,656	2,745	2,838	2,933	3,032
6.6	1,878	1,941	2,006	2,073	2,142	2,213	2,287	2,364	2,443	2,524	2,609	2,696	2,786	2,879	2,975	3,075
6.7	1,913	1,976	2,042	2,109	2,179	2,251	2,326	2,403	2,482	2,564	2,649	2,737	2,827	2,921	3,018	3,117
6.8	1,949	2,012	2,078	2,147	2,217	2,290	2,365	2,442	2,522	2,605	2,690	2,778	2,869	2,964	3,061	3,161
6.9	1,985	2,049	2,116	2,184	2,255	2,329	2,404	2,482	2,563	2,646	2,732	2,821	2,912	3,007	3,104	3,205
7.0	2,022	2,087	2,154	2,223	2,295	2,368	2,444	2,523	2,604	2,688	2,774	2,863	2,955	3,050	3,149	3,250
7.1	2,059	2,125	2,193	2,262	2,334	2,409	2,485	2,564	2,646	2,730	2,817	2,907	2,999	3,095	3,193	3,295
7.2	2,098	2,164	2,232	2,302	2,375	2,450	2,527	2,607	2,689	2,773	2,861	2,951	3,044	3,140	3,239	3,341
7.3	2,137	2,203	2,272	2,343	2,416	2,491	2,569	2,649	2,732	2,817	2,905	2,996	3,089	3,186	3,285	3,388
7.4	2,176	2,244	2,313	2,384	2,458	2,534	2,612	2,693	2,776	2,862	2,950	3,041	3,135	3,232	3,332	3,435
7.5	2,217	2,265	2,354	2,426	2,501	2,577	2,656	2,737	2,821	2,907	2,996	3,088	3,182	3,279	3,380	3,483
7.6	2,258	2,326	2,397	2,469	2,544	2,621	2,700	2,782	2,866	2,953	3,042	3,134	3,229	3,327	3,428	3,531
7.7	2,300	2,369	2,440	2,513	2,588	2,666	2,746	2,828	2,912	3,000	3,090	3,182	3,277	3,376	3,477	3,581
7.8	2,343	2,412	2,484	2,557	2,633	2,711	2,792	2,874	2,959	3,047	3,137	3,230	3,326	3,425	3,526	3,631
7.9	2,386	2,456	2,528	2,603	2,679	2,757	2,838	2,921	3,007	3,095	3,186	3,279	3,376	3,475	3,576	3,681
8.0	2,431	2,501	2,574	2,649	2,725	2,804	2,886	2,969	3,056	3,144	3,235	3,329	3,426	3,525	3,627	3,733
8.1	2,476	2,547	2,620	2,695	2,773	2,852	2,934	3,018	3,105	3,194	3,286	3,380	3,477	3,577	3,679	3,785
8.2	2,522	2,594	2,667	2,743	2,821	2,901	2,983	3,068	3,155	3,244	3,336	3,431	3,529	3,629	3,732	3,838
8.3	2,569	2,641	2,715	2,791	2,870	2,950	3,033	3,118	3,206	3,296	3,388	3,483	3,581	3,682	3,785	3,891
8.4	2,617	2,689	2,764	2,841	2,920	3,001	3,084	3,169	3,257	3,348	3,441	3,536	3,634	3,735	3,839	3,945
8.5	2,665	2,739	2,814	2,891	2,970	3,052	3,135	3,221	3,310	3,401	3,494	3,590	3,688	3,790	3,894	4,000
8.6	2,715	2,789	2,864	2,942	3,022	3,104	3,188	3,274	3,363	3,454	3,548	3,644	3,743	3,845	3,949	4,056
8.7	2,765	2,840	2,916	2,994	3,074	3,157	3,241	3,328	3,417	3,509	3,603	3,700	3,799	3,901	4,005	4,113
8.8	2,817	2,892	2,968	3,047	3,128	3,210	3,295	3,383	3,472	3,565	3,659	3,756	3,855	3,958	4,063	4,170
8.9	2,869	2,944	3,021	3,101	3,182	3,265	3,351	3,438	3,528	3,621	3,716	3,813	3,913	4,015	4,120	4,228
9.0	2,923	2,998	3,076	3,155	3,237	3,321	3,407	3,495	3,585	3,678	3,773	3,871	3,971	4,074	4,179	4,287
9.1	2,977	3,053	3,131	3,211	3,293	3,377	3,464	3,552	3,643	3,736	3,832	3,930	4,030	4,133	4,239	4,347
9.2	3,032	3,109	3,187	3,268	3,350	3,435	3,522	3,611	3,702	3,795	3,891	3,989	4,090	4,193	4,299	4,408
9.3	3,089	3,166	3,245	3,326	3,409	3,494	3,581	3,670	3,761	3,855	3,951	4,050	4,151	4,254	4,361	4,469
9.4	3,146	3,224	3,303	3,384	3,468	3,553	3,641	3,738	3,822	3,916	4,013	4,111	4,213	4,316	4,423	4,532
9.5	3,205	3,283	3,362	3,444	3,528	3,614	3,701	3,791	3,884	3,978	4,075	4,174	4,275	4,379	4,486	4,595
9.6	3,264	3,343	3,423	3,505	3,589	3,675	3,763	3,854	3,946	4,041	4,138	4,237	4,339	4,443	4,550	4,659
9.7	3,325	3,404	3,484	3,567	3,651	3,738	3,826	3,917	4,010	4,105	4,202	4,302	4,404	4,508	4,615	4,724
9.8	3,387	3,466	3,547	3,630	3,715	3,802	3,890	3,981	4,074	4,170	4,267	4,367	4,469	4,573	4,680	4,790
9.9	3,450	3,529	3,611	3,694	3,779	3,866	3,956	4,047	4,140	4,236	4,333	4,433	4,536	4,640	4,747	4,857
10.0	3,514	3,594	3,676	3,759	3,845	3,932	4,022	4,113	4,207	4,303	4,400	4,501	4,603	4,708	4,815	4,924

8.3. ABNORMAL FETAL GROWTH

- Fetal growth is considered abnormal when the newborn's weight is below or above the 10th percentile of mean weight for gestation.

- This definition of abnormal growth represents only a very crude definition, since many clearly growth-retarded or macrosomic infants will still fall within normal statistical parameters.

- Because normal growth is genetically and socioeconomically defined, at least theoretically each geographic area should establish its own normal growth curve.

8.3.1. Intrauterine Growth Retardation

Intrauterine growth retardation (IUGR) is defined as a fetus's growth parameter within or below the 10th percentile of the mean. Further definitions subdivide IUGR into symmetric and asymmetric IUGR:

- *Symmetric IUGR* is defined as symmetric growth retardation of all parameters used in sonographic evaluation of the fetus and usually represents a very early existing insult to the fetus (see Fig. 8.3.1).

  1. This classification represents a minority of IUGR cases, with asymmetric IUGR representing the majority.

  2. Symmetric IUGR is significantly more difficult to diagnose than asymmetric IUGR because of the difficulty in making a differential diagnosis on the basis of false dates. Furthermore, the *head/abdomen (H/A) ratio* will generally be normal.

  3. Representing an early insult to the fetus, symmetric IUGR is primarily associated with the following disorders:
     o Congenital and chromosomal abnormalities
     o Fetal viral diseases
     o Severe maternal medical problems

  4. The sonographic diagnosis is made only when there is considerable clinical suspicion, relying on the following sonographic findings:
     o Small-for-date growth parameters including BPD, HC, and AC
     o Normal H/A ratio

- *Asymmetric IUGR* represents a later insult to the fetus. Consequently, it will become clinically apparent at 26–30 weeks only.

  1. This classification represents the majority of IUGR cases.

  2. The sonographic diagnosis of asymmetric IUGR is significantly easier than that of symmetric IUGR as a clear discrepancy between growth parameters will become apparent on serial scans.

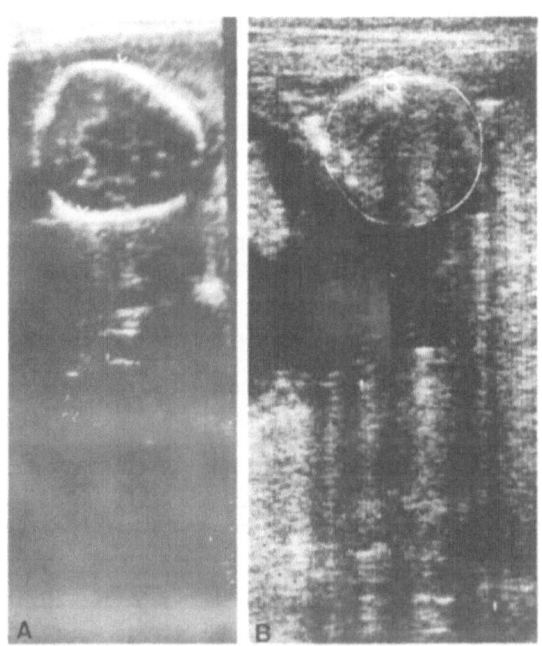

FIG. 8.3.1. SYMMETRICAL INTRAUTERINE GROWTH RETARDATION

A 27-week gestation with symmetric IUGR. (A) Biparietal diameter (BPD) compatible with 22 weeks. (B) Abdominal circumference (AC) compatible with 20 weeks. Spine (S).

3. In principle, a series of events have been described as characteristic of an asymmetric IUGR situation[6]:

    o   Increasing oligohydramnios (see Fig. 8.3.2)
    o   Decrease in body mass, which will result in an inappropriate H/A ratio (HC/AC) (see Fig. 8.3.3 and Table 8.3.1) as a head-sparing effect will allow the fetal head to continue normal growth except in the most severe cases
    o   Enhanced placental maturation (see Fig. 8.3.2)
    o   Normal growth of long bones such as the femur, which is affected in only the most severe cases, (therefore confirmation of normal femur length (FL) in conjunction with a decrease in AC will aid in the diagnosis of IUGR)

4. Conditions predisposing to asymmetric IUGR are listed in Fig. 8.1.3.

5. Accurate estimation of amniotic fluid volumes with real-time ultrasonography is impossible and has to be restricted to estimations based on clinical experience of the sonographer.

6. Once IUGR is suspected on the basis of sonographic evaluation, a routine sonographic follow-up every 2 weeks is recommended. In cases of symmetric IUGR, a detailed investigation of the fetus to rule out any major chromosomal and/or congenital abnormality may be indicated. This workup may include genetic amniocentesis (see Chapter 6), evaluation of alpha-fetoprotein (see Chapter 17) and a level II sonogram or target organ imaging (see Chapter 17).

TABLE 8.3.1.

Nomogram for H/A Ratio

Menstrual age (weeks)	H/A circumference ratio		
	5th Centile	Mean	95th Centile
13–14	1.14	1.23	1.31
15–16	1.05	1.22	1.39
17–18	1.07	1.18	1.29
19–20	1.09	1.18	1.26
21–22	1.06	1.15	1.25
23–24	1.05	1.13	1.21
25–26	1.04	1.13	1.22
27–28	1.05	1.13	1.22
29–30	0.99	1.10	1.21
31–32	0.96	1.07	1.17
33–34	0.96	1.04	1.11
35–36	0.93	1.02	1.11
37–38	0.92	0.98	1.05
39–40	0.87	0.97	1.06
41–42	0.93	0.96	1.00

[a]From Campbell, *et al.*[7]

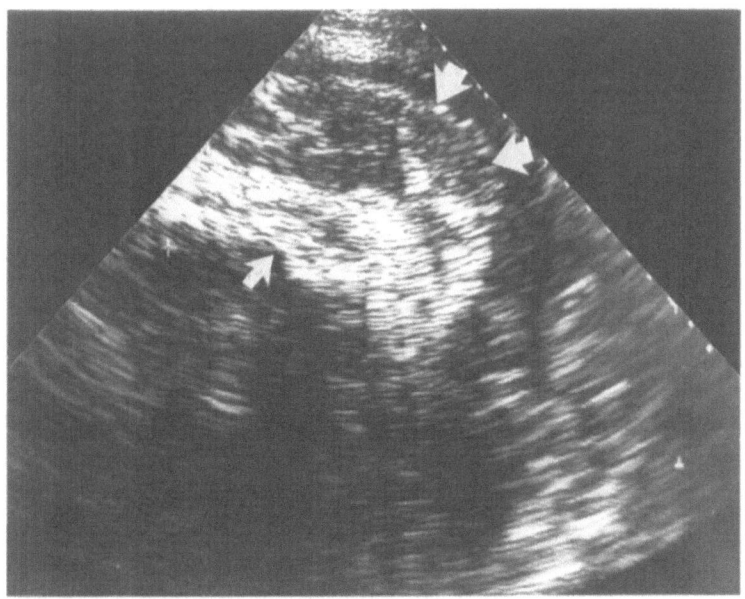

FIG. 8.3.2. PLACENTAL AND AMNIOTIC FLUID FINDINGS IN INTRAUTERINE GROWTH RETARDATION

Large arrows point to the calcified areas of cotyledons in a grade III placenta. Note the absence of amniotic fluid. Fetal part (small arrow).

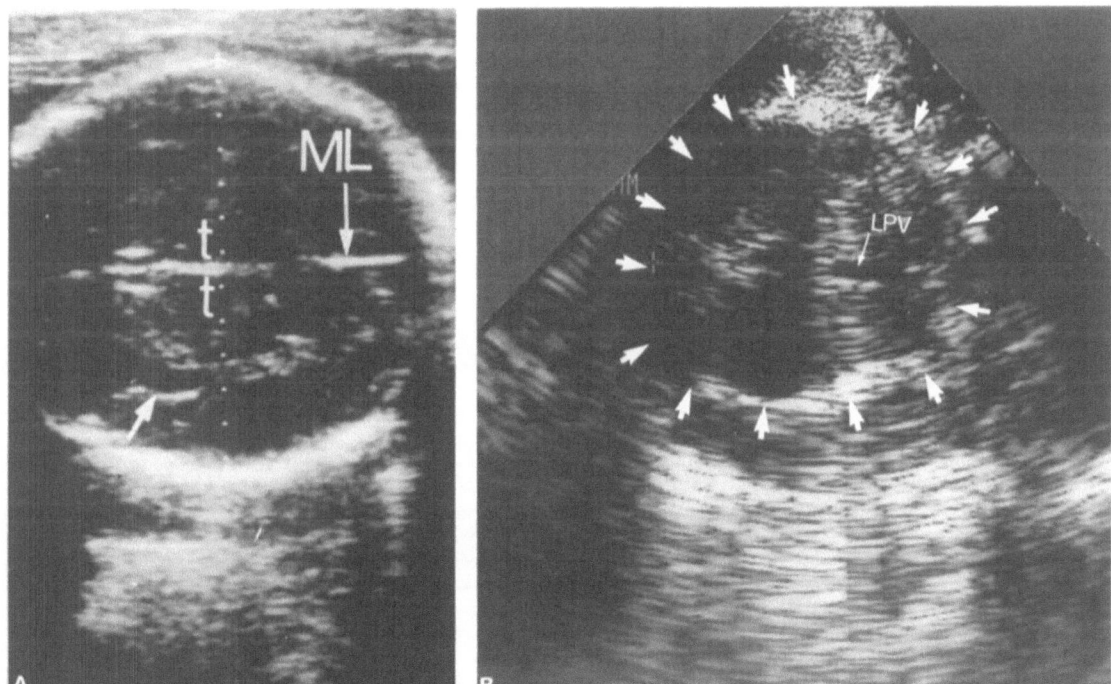

FIG. 8.3.3. NORMAL BIPARIETAL DIAMETER AND SMALL ABDOMINAL CIRCUMFERENCE IN ASYMMETRIC IUGR

Size discrepancy between a normal BPD (A) and small AC (B) in asymmetric IUGR. Note the minimal amount of amniotic fluid surrounding the AC. (A) midline (ML), thalami (t), insula (arrow). (B) AC (arrows), left portal vein (LPV).

7. Some investigators recommend a *biophysical profile* for the evaluation of fetal well-being in conjunction with IUGR (and also normal growth).[8,9] In addition to widely used parameters for the assessment of fetal antepartum well-being, such as nonstress testing (NST) and contraction stress testing (OCT), these investigators added several sonographically determined parameters indicative of fetal well-being:

o Fetal breathing movements
o Fetal movements
o Fetal tone
o Amniotic fluid volume
o Placental grading

Criteria for scoring of a biophysical profile are presented in Table 8.3.2.

REFERENCES

6. DeVore GR, Hobbins JC: Fetal growth and development: The diagnosis of intrauterine growth retardation, in Hobbins JC (ed): *Diagnostic Ultrasound in Obstetrics,* New York, Churchill Livingstone, 1979, p 81.
7. Campbell S: Ultrasound measurement of the fetal head to abdomen circumference ratio in assessment of growth retardation. *Br J Gynaecol* 1977;84:165.
8. Manning F, Platt LD, Sipos L: Antepartum fetal evaluation. Development of a fetal biophysical profile. *Am J Obstet Gynecol.* 1980;136:787.
9. Vintzileos AM, Campbell WA, Ingardia CT, et al: The fetal biophysical profile and its predictive value. *Obstet Gynecol* 1983;62:271.

TABLE 8.3.2

Criteria for Scoring the Biophysical Profile

Nonstress test
  Score 2 (NST 2): Five or more accelerations of at least 15 bpm in amplitude and at least 15-sec duration associated with fetal movements in a 20-min period
  Score 1 (NST 1): Two to four accelerations of at least 15 bpm in amplitude and at least 15-sec duration associated with fetal movements in a 20-min period
Fetal movements
  Score 2 (FM 2): At least three gross (trunk and limbs) episodes of fetal movements within 30 min. Simultaneous limb and trunk movements
  Score 1 (FM 1): One or two fetal movements within 30 min
  Score 0 (FM 0): Absence of fetal movements within 30 min
Fetal breathing movements
  Score 2 (FBM 2): At least one episode of fetal breathing of at least 60-sec duration within a 30-min observation period
  Score 1 (FBM 1): At least one episode of fetal breathing lasting 30–60 sec within a 30 min period
  Score 0 (FBM 0): Absence of fetal breathing or breathing lasting less than 30 sec within a 30-min period
Fetal tone
  Score 2 (FT 2): At least one episode of extension of extremities with return to position of flexion and also one episode of extension of spine with return to position of flexion
  Score 1 (FT 1): At least one episode of extension of extremities with return to position of flexion, or one episode of extension of spine with return to position of flexion
  Score 0 (FT 0): Extremities in extension; fetal movements not followed by return to flexion; open hand
Amniotic fluid volume
  Score 2 (AF 2): Fluid evident throughout the uterine cavity; a pocket that measures ≥2 cm in vertical diameter
  Score 1 (AF 1): A pocket that measures <2 cm but >1 cm in vertical diameter
  Score 0 (AF 0): Crowding of fetal small parts; largest pocket <1 cm in vertical diameter
Placenta grading
  Score 2 (PL 2): Placenta grading 0, 1, or 2
  Score 1 (PL 1): Placenta posterior difficult to evaluate
  Score 0 (PL 0): Placenta grading 3

NST, nonstress test; FHR, fetal heart rate; bpm, beats per minute; FM, fetal movements; FT, fetal tone; AF, amniotic fluid; PL, placenta grading; FBM, fetal breathing movements.
Adapted from Vintzileos et al.[9]

8.3.2. Fetal Macrosomia

- Macrosomia is suspected sonographically when individual fetal growth parameters are found to be within or above the upper 10th percentile of the mean.

- Classically, macrosomia is associated with maternal diabetes (milder disease) (see Figs. 8.3.4 and 8.3.5). (See detailed discussion in Chapter 9.)

- Other instances of large fetuses can be found with immunologic and nonimmunologic fetal hydrops. (See full discussion in Chapters 10 and 11.)

- Larger-than-normal placentae are found in most instances of *hyperplacentosis*, which may occur in several conditions:

  Diabetes mellitus
  Syphilis
  Erythroblastosis fetalis
  Nonimmunologic hydrops
  Multiple birth
  Preclinical stages of EPH gestosis (preeclampsia)

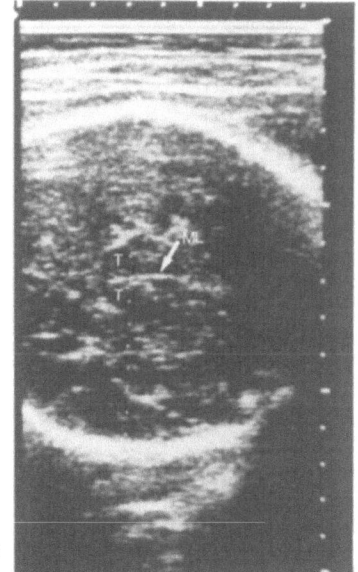

FIG. 8.3.4. LARGE-FOR-DATE BIPARIETAL DIAMETER IN DIABETIC PREGNANCY

Transverse scan through the fetal head at 32 weeks gestation demonstrating a large BPD for the gestational age: (BPD, 9.3 cm). Midline (ML), thalami (T).

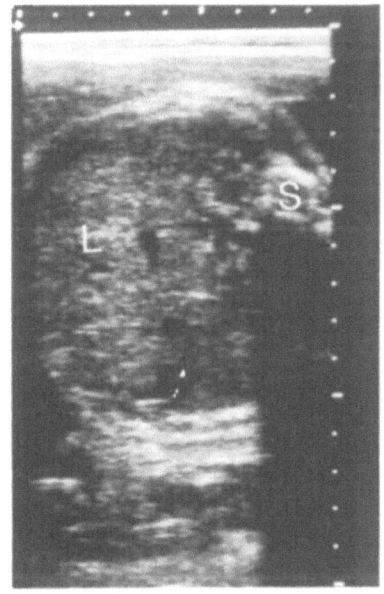

FIG. 8.3.5. LARGE-FOR-DATE ABDOMINAL CIRCUMFERENCE IN DIABETIC PREGNANCY

Transverse sonogram of the fetal abdomen in a macrosomic fetus. Difficulty is encountered in fitting the entire abdomen on the screen in the large-for-gestational age (LGA) fetus. Spine (S), liver (L). (Transducers with larger fields of view can accommodate this technical difficulty.)

Chapter 9
Diabetes Mellitus

Diabetes mellitus is clinically relevant to obstetric sonography because the following clinical occurrences in the fetus can be monitored sonographically.

9.1. FETAL MACROSOMIA

- Fetal macrosomia is clearly associated with the milder forms of maternal diabetes mellitus (largely classes A and B).

- The sonographic diagnosis is made by the demonstration of several findings:
    - Polyhydramnios (see Fig. 9.1.1)
    - Placentomegaly (hyperplacentosis) (see Fig. 9.1.2)
    - Large individual growth parameters
    - Small head/abdomen (H/A) ratio
    - Sonographic evidence of skin thickening, seen at times as a double contour
    - See also Figs. 9.1.3 and 9.1.4.

9.2. FETAL IUGR

- Fetal intrauterine growth retardation (IUGR) associated with maternal diabetes mellitus occurs primarily in association with more severe maternal disease (classes C–R).

- IUGR is usually asymmetric and presents as discussed in Section 8.3.1.

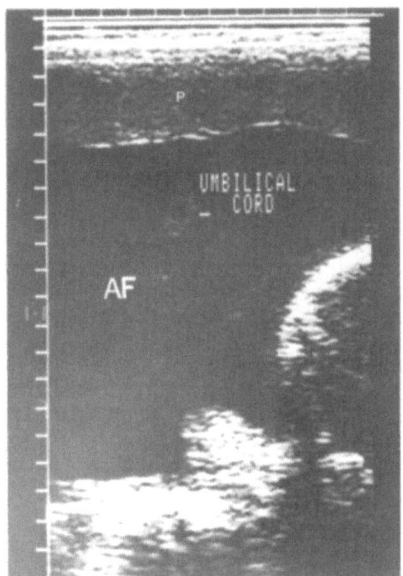

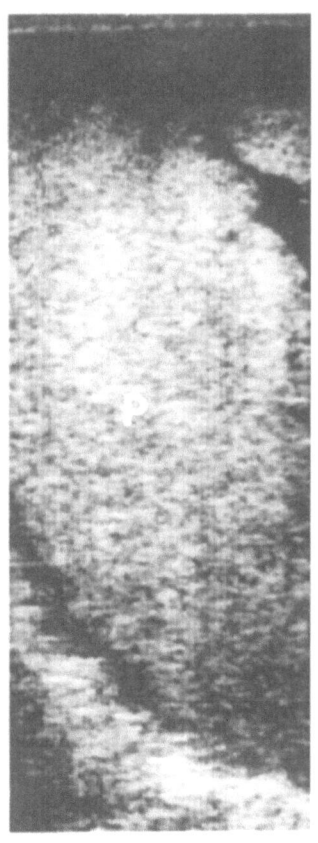

FIG. 9.1.1. POLYHYDRAM-NIOS IN DIABETIC PREG-NANCY Oblique scan demonstrating severe polyhydramnios (AF) in a diabetic pregnancy at 32 weeks. Placenta (P).

FIG. 9.1.2. ENLARGED PLACENTA IN DIABETIC PREGNANCY Longitudinal scan demonstrating an enlarged fundal placenta (P).

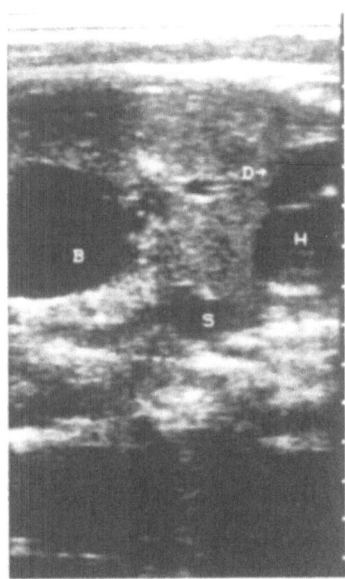

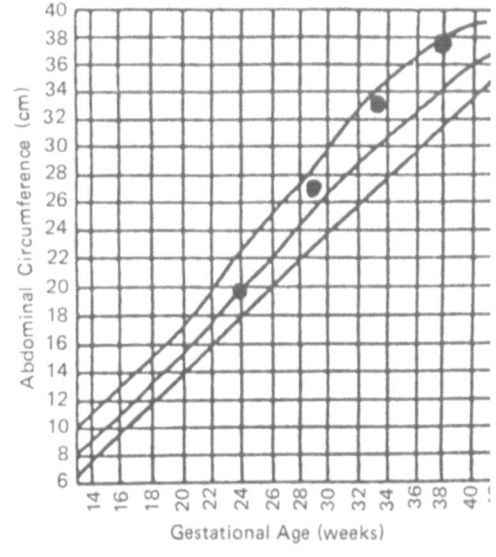

FIG. 9.1.3. ENLARGED FETAL BLADDER IN FETUS OF DIABETIC PREGNANCY Longitudinal scan demonstrating an enlarged fetal bladder (B). Diaphragm (D), heart (H), stomach (S).

FIG. 9.1.4. SERIAL BIPARIETAL AND ABDOMINAL CIRCUMFERENCE MEASUREMENTS OF A MAC-ROSOMIC DIABETIC PREGNANCY Graphic demonstration of serial sonograms with an increase in abdominal circumference (AC) from the 50th to the 95th percentile.

9.3. CONGENITAL ANOMALIES

- Congenital anomalies are increased in diabetic pregnancies.[1]

- The most frequent major congenital abnormalities associated with DM are the following:

  o Cardiovascular abnormalities
  o Neural tube defects (particularly sacral agenesis)
  o Renal abnormalities
  o Skeletal abnormalities
  o Gastrointestinal abnormalities

- Consequently, a level II sonogram (target organ imaging) should be performed in all diabetic pregnancies, classes B–R. (For further detail, see Chapter 17.)

REFERENCE

1. Simpson JL, Elias S, Martin AO, et al: Diabetes in pregnancy. Northwestern University series (1970–1981). *Am J Obstet Gynecol* 1983;146:263.

9.4. DELIVERY OF THE DIABETIC PREGNANCY

- Timed delivery in diabetic pregnancies frequently becomes a clinical necessity. Consequently, every diabetic pregnancy requires most accurate gestational dating as well as fetal weight estimation.

- Serial sonography therefore represents a cornerstone of modern management of the diabetic pregnancy.

Chapter 10
Erythroblastosis Fetalis and Other Immune Sensitizations of the Fetus

- Only rarely is the diagnosis of erythroblastosis fetalis (EF) made sonographically. Immune sensitization of the fetus should, however, always be considered when hydropic signs are noted sonographically.

- The sonographic relevance to the immune sensitization of the fetus lies in the following issues.

10.1. AMNIOCENTESIS

- Once maternal antibodies have been detected, serial amniotic fluid studies are performed to evaluate the severity of fetal disease.

- These amniocenteses should be performed under sonographic control, as described in detail in Chapter 6.

- Recently, it has been suggested that the severity of fetal involvement may be evaluated sonographically, thereby reducing the need for amniocentesis.[1]

10.2. FETAL ASSESSMENT

- Fetal involvement (anemia) will correlate to the severity of fetal hydrops. The more affected the fetus, the more hydropic it will present sonographically.

- The sonographic picture of hydrops is characterized by the following findings:

    o Placentomegaly (hyperplacentosis) (see Fig. 9.1.2)
    o Fetal hepatomegaly (see Fig. 10.2.4)
    o Fetal ascites (see Figs. 10.2.1 and 10.2.3)
    o Fetal pericardial/pleural effusions
    o Fetal scalp edema
    o Fetal peripheral skin edema (e.g., facial edema) (see Fig. 10.2.2)
    o Scrotal edema
    o Enlarged umbilical vein diameter[2]

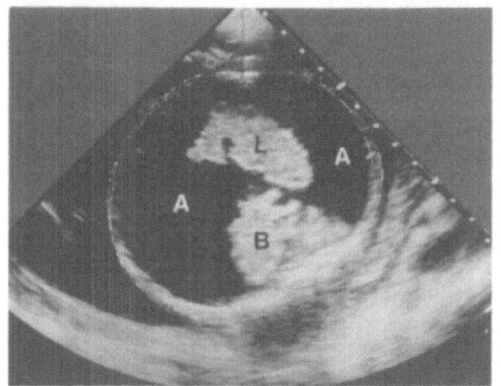

FIG. 10.2.1. ASCITES IN HYDROPIC FETUS DUE TO Rh-NEGATIVE DISEASE Transverse scan through the fetal abdomen demonstrating massive ascites (A) with fetal liver (L) and bowel loops (B) floating free. (Trace marks are also visualized, indicating the AC).

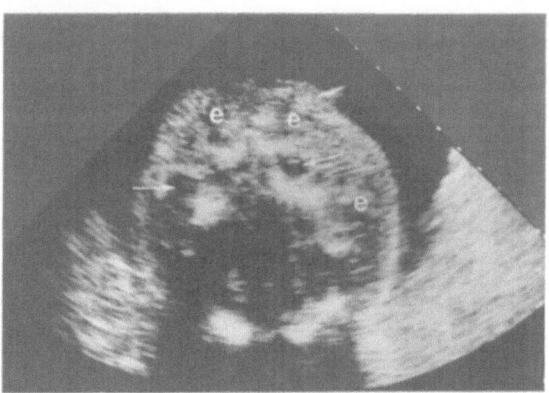

FIG. 10.2.2. SEVERE FACIAL EDEMA IN HYDROPIC INFANT DUE TO Rh-NEGATIVE DISEASE Transverse sector scan of the fetal head in an occiptal posterior (face-up) position, demonstrating facial edema (e). Orbits (arrows).

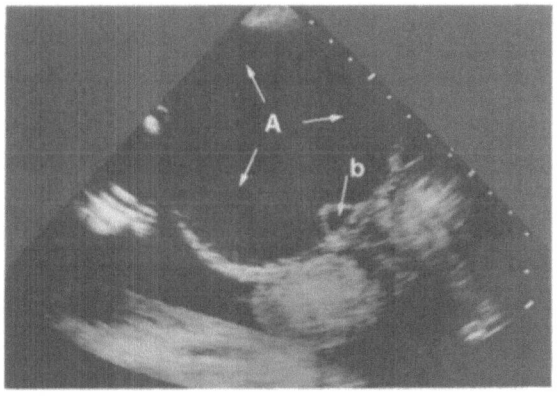

FIG. 10.2.3. PELVIC ASCITES IN HYDROPIC FETUS DUE TO Rh-NEGATIVE DISEASE Transverse sector scan of the fetal pelvis demonstrating massive ascites (A) and the normal fetal bladder (b).

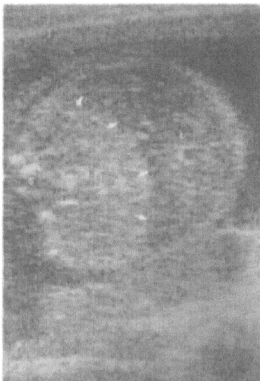

FIG. 10.2.4. HEPATOMEGALY IN Rh-NEGATIVE SENSITIZED FETUS Transverse scan through the fetal abdomen illustrating an enlarged liver (L). Note the enhanced interface (arrows) between the liver parenchyma and bowel (B). Spine (s). From Grannum et al.[4]

10.3. INTRAUTERINE TRANSFUSION AND PARACENTESIS

- Sonography is now widely used in the controlled insertion of the transfusion needle into the fetal abdomen.[3]

- Similarly, extreme cases of fetal ascites have been decompressed before delivery of the fetus, using sonographically directed paracentesis.

REFERENCES

1. Platt LD, Manning FA: Real-time ultrasound in special procedures. *Clin Diagn Ultrasound* 1979;3:165.
2. DeVore GR, Mayden KL, Tortora M, et al: Dilation of the umbilical vein in Rhesus hemolytic anemia: A predictor of severe disease. *Am J Obstet Gynecol* 1981;141:464.
3. Hobbins JC, Davis CD, Webster T: A new technique utilizing ultrasound to aid in intrauterine transfusion. *J Clin Ultrasound* 1976;4:135.
4. Grannum PAT, Tortora M, Mayden KL, Taylor KJW: Obstetrical Ultrasound, in Taylor KJW (ed): *Atlas of Ultrasonography*, ed 2. New York, Churchill Livingstone, 1985.

Chapter 11
Nonimmunologic
Hydrops

The sonographic presentation of nonimmunologic hydrops (see Fig. 11.1.1) is identical to that of immunologic hydrops. Once immunologic causes of hydrops have been excluded, the following conditions associated with nonimmunologic hydrops or isolated fetal ascites have to be ruled out.

1. FETAL ANEMIA

2. FETAL CARDIAC ABNORMALITIES

   - Congestive heart failure due to:
     o Supraventricular tachycardia
     o Complete heart block

   - Structural congenital heart disease:
     o Ebstein's anomaly
     o Hypoplastic left heart syndrome

3. RENAL ANOMALIES

4. CONGENITAL INFECTIONS

   - Syphilis
   - Toxoplasmosis
   - Cytomegalovirus

5. PULMONARY MALFORMATIONS

6. FETAL BOWEL VOLVULUS

7. FETAL MECONIUM PERITONITIS

8. OBSTRUCTION OR ABSENCE OF THORACIC DUCT

9. CYSTIC HYGROMA OF THE FETUS

   - Sonographically, a level II sonogram (target organ imaging) and intrauterine echocardiography are indicated in all instances of nonimmunologic hydrops.
   - Fetal diagnostic or therapeutic paracentesis is possible under sonographic control.

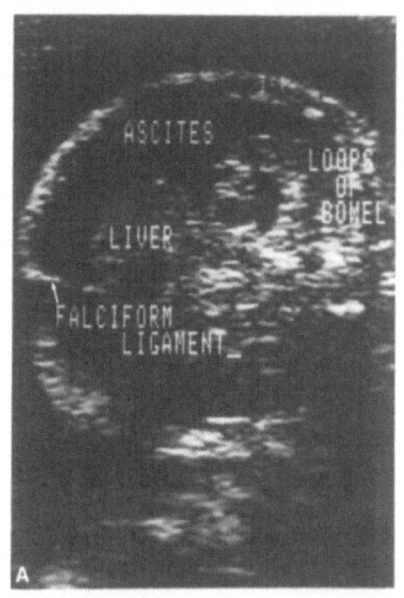

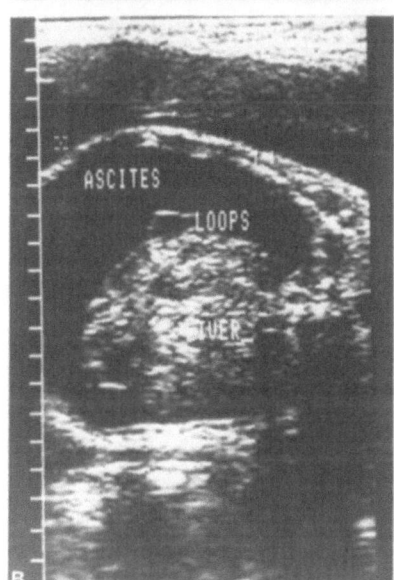

FIG. 11.1.1. NONIMMUNOLOGIC HYDROPS

(A) Transverse scan through the fetal abdomen illustrating ascites in a patient with nonimmunologic hydrops.

(B) Longitudinal scan in same patient illustrating nonimmunologic hydrops.

Chapter 12
Multiple Pregnancies

12.1. NORMALS

- Despite increasing use of obstetric sonography, multiple pregnancies remain frequently undiagnosed until delivery.

- Routine obstetric scanning therefore should always include a sweep from lateral to lateral border of the uterus and from symphysis to the uterine fundus.

- Once a multiple gestation is diagnosed beyond the first trimester, the accurate definition of individual fetuses is essential. Numbers of heads, fetal bodies, and limbs have to be clearly established. Errors in reported number of fetuses in a multiple pregnancy are still rather frequent.[1]

- Several sonographic factors need to be identified with multiple gestations:
  - Fetal positions
  - Fetal membranes to determine number of fetal sacs (see Fig. 12.1.1)
  - Number of placentae and localization
  - Amniotic fluid estimate for each sac
  - Growth parameters for each fetus
  - Presence of normal anatomy for each fetus

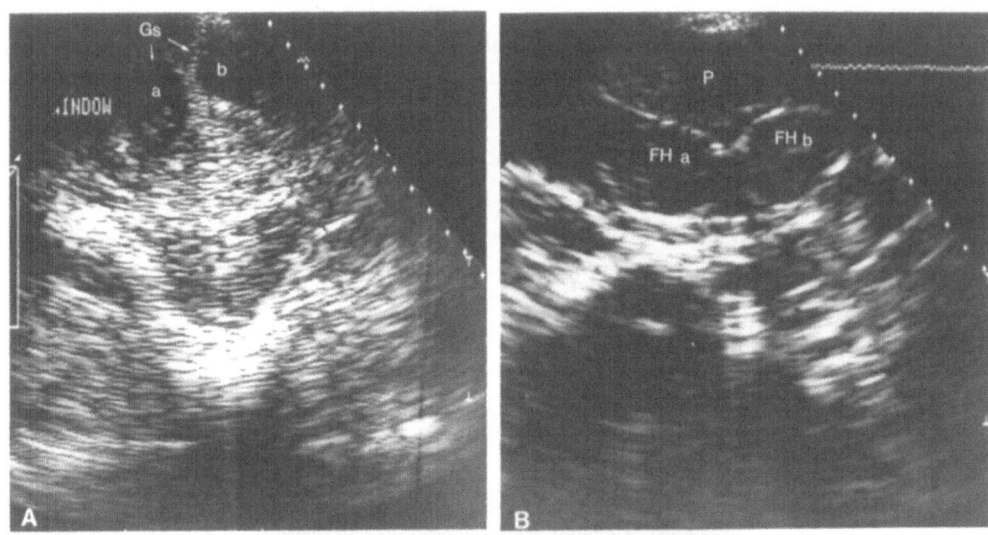

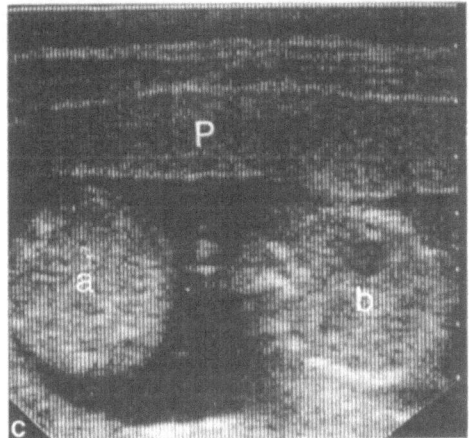

FIG. 12.1.1. TWIN GESTATIONS

(A) Twin gestational sacs (a and b) at 5–7 weeks gestation.

(B) Twin fetal heads (A and B) in a transverse section at approximately the level of the biparietal diameter (BPD) at 14–15 weeks. Placenta (P).

(C) Twin fetal bodies (a and b) in a transverse section at 17–18 weeks gestation. Placenta (P).

- Growth curves for multiple gestations vary from singleton growth curves. This must be taken into account in the assessment of multiple gestations (see Fig. 12.1.2).

- Serial sonography on a monthly basis is recommended for multiple pregnancies.

- When amniocentesis is indicated in a multiple pregnancy, attempts can be made to identify the individual sacs by sonographic visualization of membranes, thereby facilitating proper needle placement (see Fig. 12.1.3).

REFERENCES

1. Gleicher N, Olaya B, Hercule J, et al: The diagnosis of multiple gestation. *Diagn Gynecol Obstet* 1983;4:223.
2. Leveno KJ, Santos-Ramos R, Duenhoelter JH, et al: Sonar cephalometry in twins: A table of biparietal diameters for normal twin fetuses and a comparison with singletons. *Am J Obstet Gynecol* 1979;135:727.
3. Grannum PAT, Tortora M, Mayden KL, Taylor KJW: Obstetrical ultrasound, in Taylor KJW (ed): *Atlas of Ultrasonography*, ed 2, New York, Churchill Livingstone, 1985.

12.2. ABNORMALS

If abnormalities or discordance or both, in the growth pattern of any of the fetuses is noted, serial sonographic evaluations have to be made.

12.2.1. Intrauterine Transfusion Syndrome and Discordant Pregnancies

- Intrauterine transfusion syndrome (ITS) is characterized by the following findings:

  o Divergence of growth patterns between fetuses
  o Possible hydropic changes in larger fetus
  o Polyhydramnios in larger fetal compartment
  o Oligohydramnios in smaller fetal compartment
  o Enhanced placental maturation in smaller fetal compartment
  o Enhanced fetal maturation in smaller fetal compartment

- ITS is largely restricted to monozygotic twins. Consequently, the sonographic visualization of membranes, representing two separate sacs, statistically mitigates against ITS.

- Once intrauterine growth retardation (IUGR) is suspected in one or more fetuses, management as outlined in Section 8.3 is to be followed.

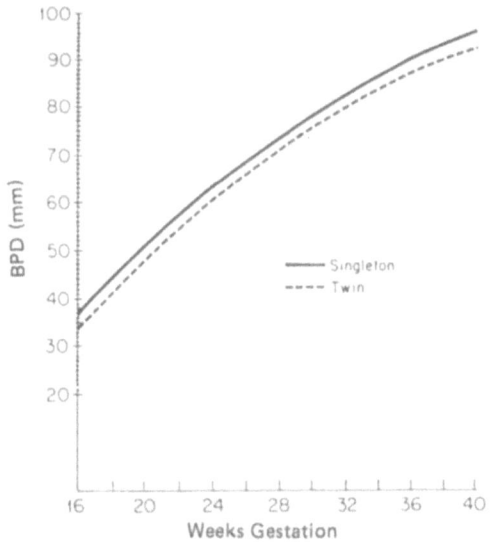

FIG. 12.1.2. TWIN GROWTH CURVES

Smoothed mean twin (- - -) and singleton (————) biparietal diameters (BPD) between 16 and 40 weeks gestation. Smoothing was done by using polynomial regression equations.
Equation for twins[2]:

$$\text{Predicted BPD} = -45.097 + 5.827 \text{ weeks} - 0.0597 \text{ (weeks)}$$

Equation for singletons[2]:

$$\text{Predicted BPD} = -39.424 + 5.694 \text{ weeks} - 0.0578 \text{ (weeks)}$$

From Leveno et al.[2]

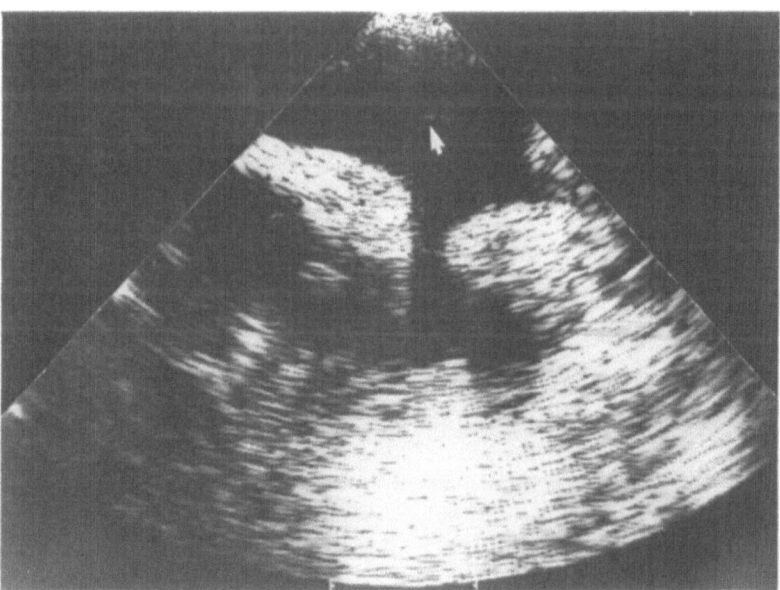

FIG. 12.1.3. MULTIPLE PREGNANCY

Sector scan demonstrating the confluence (arrow) of the three sac membranes in a triplet pregnancy.

From Gleicher et al.[1]

CHAPTER 12 • MULTIPLE PREGNANCIES

12.2.2. Conjoined Twins

The possibility of conjoined twins has to be considered once the diagnosis of twins in a symmetric presentation is made sonographically.

12.2.3. Fetus Papyraceous

This disorder represents the extreme of a discordant pregnancy situation. Sonographic diagnosis is possible at times (Fig. 12.2.1).

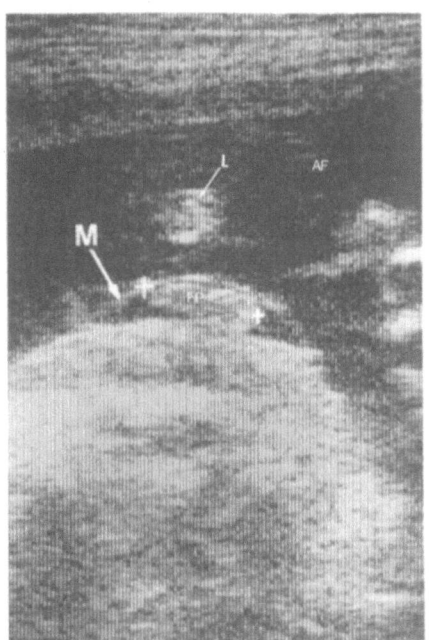

FIG. 12.2.1. FETUS PAPYRACEOUS

Longitudinal scan in a 20-week gestation illustrating a fetus papyraceous (FP).
Note the membrane (M) surrounding the fetus papyraceous. Normal amniotic fluid
(AF) and a fetal limb (L) can be identified in the other twin sac.

From Grannum et al.[3]

Chapter 13
First Trimester Bleeding

- Sonography is indicated with first trimester bleeding when a pregnancy is considered threatened. There is no indication for sonography once an abortion is completed unless incomplete abortion is a consideration. (See also Section 13.1.3.)

- Once sonography is performed for *threatened abortion,* the following differential diagnoses have to be considered:

13.1. ABNORMAL GESTATIONAL SAC

13.1.1. Empty Sac

- *Blighted ovum* represents the absence of normal contents of the gestational sac by 8 weeks gestational age (see Fig. 13.1.1).

- Normally, a *fetal pole* and *fetal circulatory pulsations* should be apparent at 6–7 weeks, but a fetal heartbeat should be definitively apparent at 9 weeks.[1] (See also Chapter 7.)

13.1.2. Separation of the Gestational Sac

- In threatened abortions, early separation of the gestational sac may occur as a sonographically fluid-filled space immediately adjacent to the sac. It is important to separate this finding from the frequently observed *implantation bleed,* which may be normal and is generally smaller in size (see Fig. 13.1.2).

- The vast majority of implantations occur high in the fundus. The sonographic visualization of a low location of the gestational sac is suspicious of separation. In some cases separation tracks can be seen.

- No gestation should be terminated due to a low position of the sac; it is only noteworthy and should be followed up.

- The normal sonographic sac is circular and smooth with a thickened border (rind appearance). Irregularly shaped sacs may indicate separation and impending abortion (see Figs. 13.1.1 and 13.1.2).

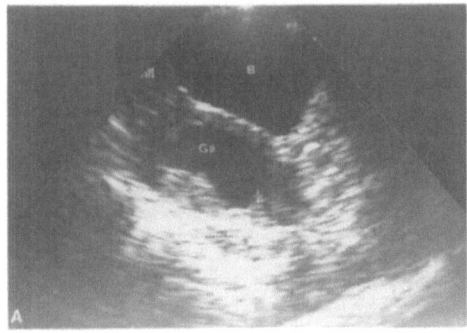 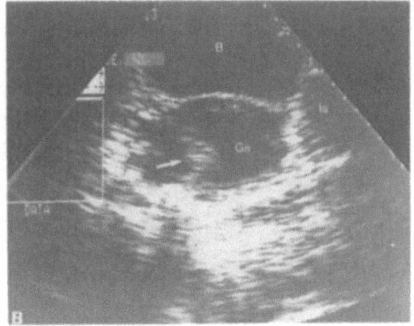

FIG. 13.1.1. BLIGHTED OVUM

Longitudinal (A) and transverse (B) sector scans demonstrating a blighted ovum (Gs) at 8–9 weeks gestation. Note the absence of internal echoes and the separation (arrow) of the sac lining. Bladder (B), iliopsoas (Is), gestational sac (Gs).

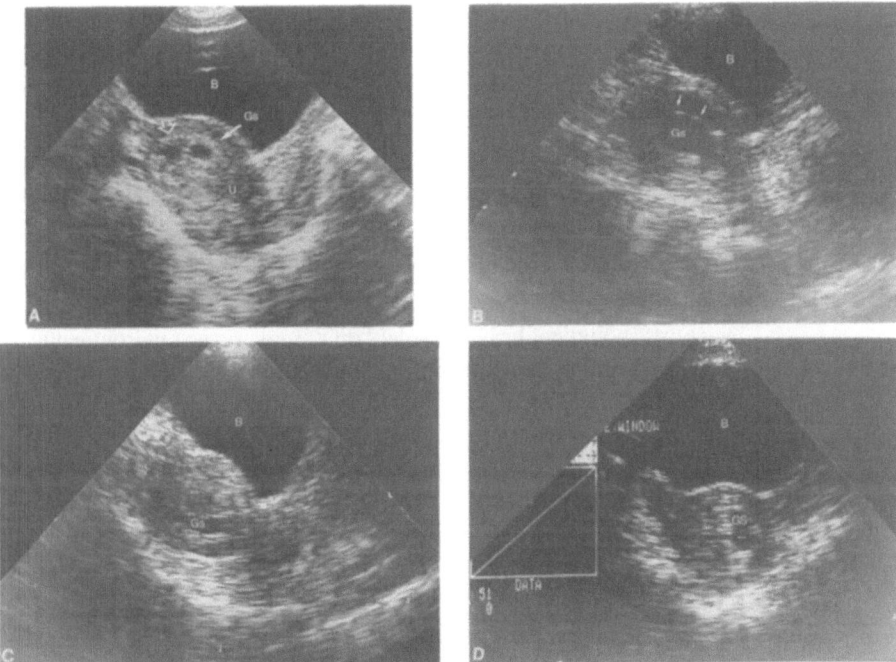

FIG. 13.1.2. ABNORMAL GESTATIONAL SACS: 4–6 WEEKS

(A) Implantation bleed (open arrow) visualized on a longitudinal scan posterior to the gestational sac (Gs). Bladder (B), uterus (U).

(B) Longitudinal sector scan demonstrating an anterior separation (arrows) of the gestational sac (Gs). Bladder (B).

(C) Longitudinal sector scan demonstrating an irregularly shaped gestational sac (Gs). Bladder (B).

(D) Transverse sector scan demonstrating an irregularly shaped sac (GS). Also shown is a break in the "rind" of the sac (arrow). Bladder (B).

13.1.3. Incomplete Abortion

This diagnosis has to be considered when echogenic patterns are noted within the uterine cavity without recognition of a gestational sac. An abnormally prominent endometrial echo complex is usually seen. In some cases individual fetal parts can be visualized (see Fig. 13.1.3).

13.1.4. Missed Abortion

This entity represents the lack of fetal heart activity in a previously confirmed live pregnancy with concomitant cessation of fetal growth.

- In all forms of abortion, fluid in the cul-de-sac may be excessive.

- It is important to remember that before 5 weeks gestation, a pregnancy is usually not diagnosed by sonographic evaluation. Extreme caution should be used in the patient with questionable or possible very early dates to avoid the possibility of a false-negative result.

- Normal gestational sacs, usually having fundal locations, are eccentric to the midline. This is an important point of differential diagnosis for the so-called *pseudo-gestational sac,* which is reported to confuse the sonographic picture in some cases of ectopic pregnancy.[2] (See Chapter 14.)

- While sonographic presentations of threatened abortions are fairly typical, interventions should not be based solely on a single scan. Environmental factors, such as fibroid tumors, may at times distort the normal picture of an early gestation, mimicking an abnormal sac (see Fig. 13.1.4).

REFERENCES

1. Jouppila P, Huhtaniemi I, Tapanainen J: Early pregnancy failure: Study by ultrasonic and hormonal methods. *Obstet Gynecol* 1980;55:42.
2. Sprit BH, O'Hara KR, Gordon L: Pseudogestational sac in ectopic pregnancy: Sonographic and pathologic correlation. *J Clin Ultrasound* 1981;9:338.

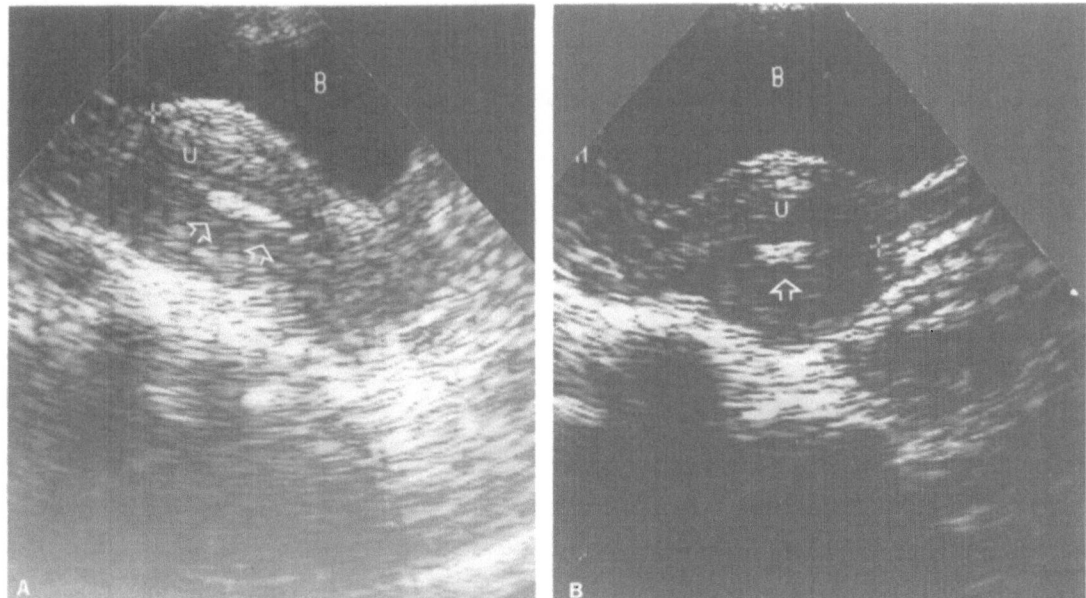

FIG. 13.1.3. INCOMPLETE ABORTION

Longitudinal (A) and transverse (B) scans of an incomplete abortion. Note the enlarged uterus and characteristically prominent endometrial echo (open arrowheads). Bladder (B), uterus (U).

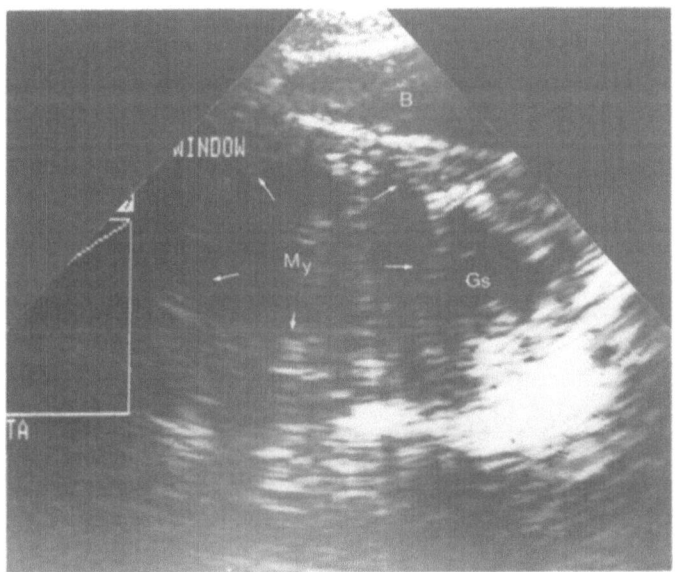

FIG. 13.1.4. ABNORMALLY SHAPED GESTATIONAL SAC

Sector scan demonstrating an abnormal-appearing gestational sac caused by fibroid tumor with normal pregnancy outcome. Note the abnormal shape of the sac. Bladder (B), myoma (My), gestational sac (Gs).

Chapter 14
Ectopic Pregnancy

- Sonography has become a cornerstone in the diagnosis of unruptured ectopic pregnancy (EP).

- Sonography is relevant for the diagnosis of EP in two aspects:

  o By exclusion of a gestational sac once a positive pregnancy test is obtained
  o Through the direct visualization of the EP[1]

- While *pseudo-gestational sacs* have been reported in cases of EP, the vast majority of cases will fail to show an intrauterine gestational sac, eccentrically located within the uterine cavity.

- Once an intrauterine gestational sac cannot be visualized with a clearly positive pregnancy test, two possibilities have to be considered:

  o The patient may be in the *critical zone* between a positive pregnancy test and first visibility of a gestational sac[2]
    OR
  o An EP is present. This is the more likely possibility once a presumptive gestational age is reached, at which a gestational sac should definitely have been visible. (See Chapters 7 and 13.)

- Sonographic findings suggestive of EP include the following:

  o Enlarged uterus
  o Absence of normal gestational sac in the uterus with positive pregnancy test
  o Excessive fluid in the cul de sac (see Section 19.2.1)
  o Adnexal mass that may vary in appearance from that of a characteristic gestational sac and/or recognition of a fetus within a complex sonographic picture (see Figs. 14.1.1 and 14.1.2)

- Most unruptured EPs can be diagnosed by sonographic evaluation.[1]

REFERENCES

1. Gleicher N, Giglia RV, Deppe G, et al: Direct diagnosis of unruptured ectopic pregnancy by real-time ultrasonography. *Obstet Gynecol* 1983;61:425.
2. Kadar N, DeVore G, Romero R, et al: The discriminatory HCG zone: Its use in the sonographic evaluation for ectopic pregnancy. *Obstet Gynecol* 1978;58:156.

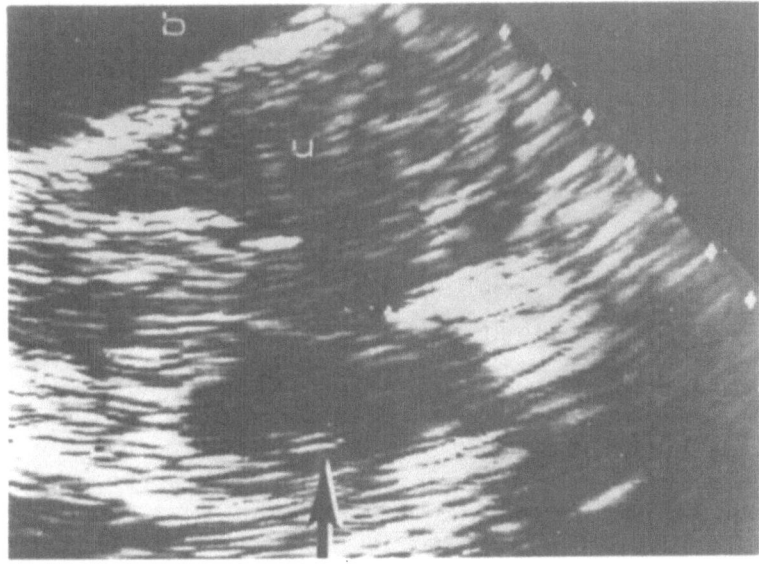

FIG. 14.1.1. UNRUPTURED TUBAL PREGNANCY

Real-time sector scan of early tubal pregnancy at approximately 8–9 weeks gestational age. A gestational sac can be seen immediately below the uterus (u), bladder (b). At the lower pole of the sac a fetus with a crown–rump length of 2.3 cm can be visualized (arrow). From Gleicher *et al.*[1]

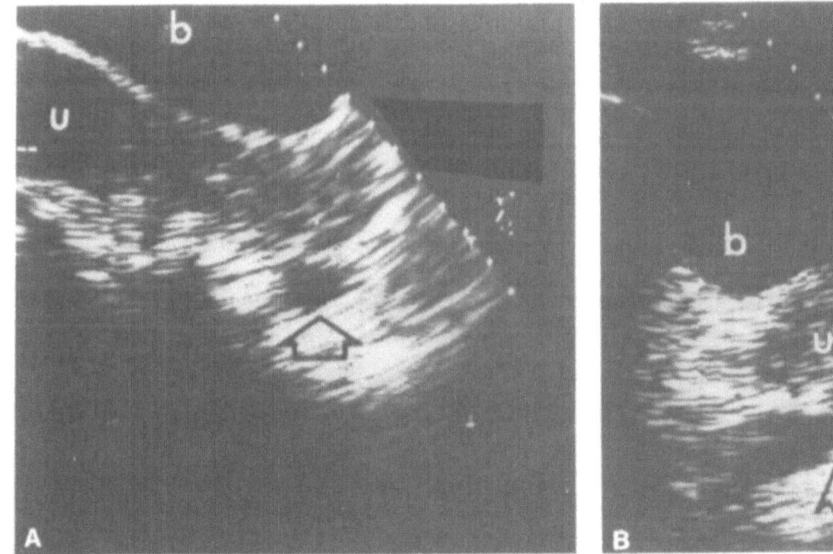
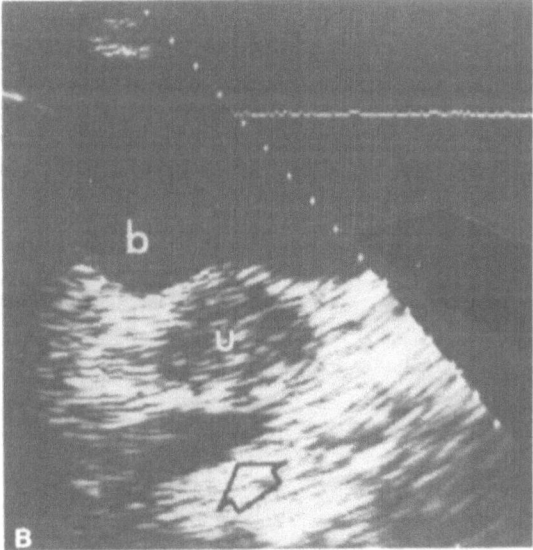

FIG. 14.1.2. RUPTURED TUBAL PREGNANCY

Longitudinal (A) and transverse (B) real-time sector scans through the pelvis. Fluid in the cul-de-sac (arrow) is demonstrated on both scans. Uterus (u), bladder (b).
From Gleicher *et al.*[1]

Chapter 15
Molar Pregnancy

- The diagnosis of molar pregnancy has been revolutionized with the advent of sonography. Few real-time sonographic patterns are as characteristic as the classic *snowstorm* pattern of a molar pregnancy as originally described with *static* scanners.

- Real-time sonography will give a slightly different sonographic appearance: Placentalike tissue fills the entire uterus with no recognizable fetal structures visible (see Fig. 15.1.1).

- The presence of a molar pregnancy should not preclude the sonographic search for a normal pregnancy. *Incomplete moles* may contain both. Furthermore, the possibility of coexistence between molar and normal pregnancy has been shown.

- Molar pregnancies are frequently accompanied by large theca–lutein cysts of the ovary that may serve as a sonographic adjunct to the diagnosis (see Section 21.2.2).

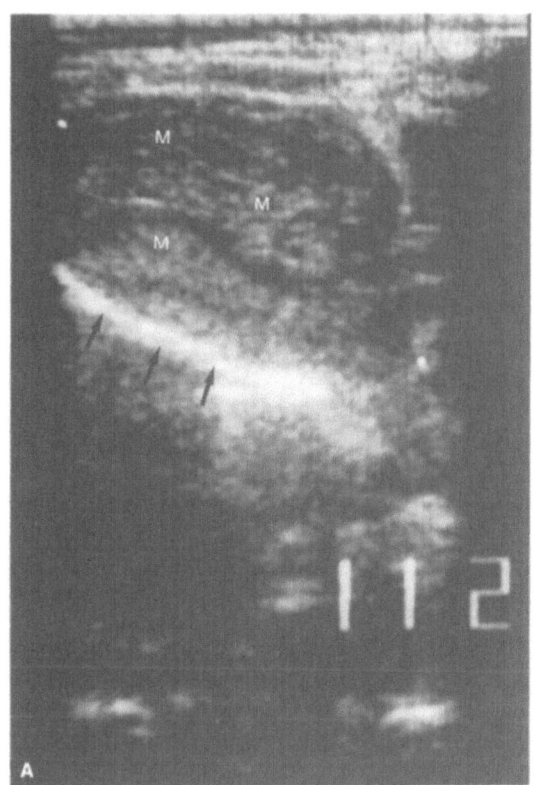

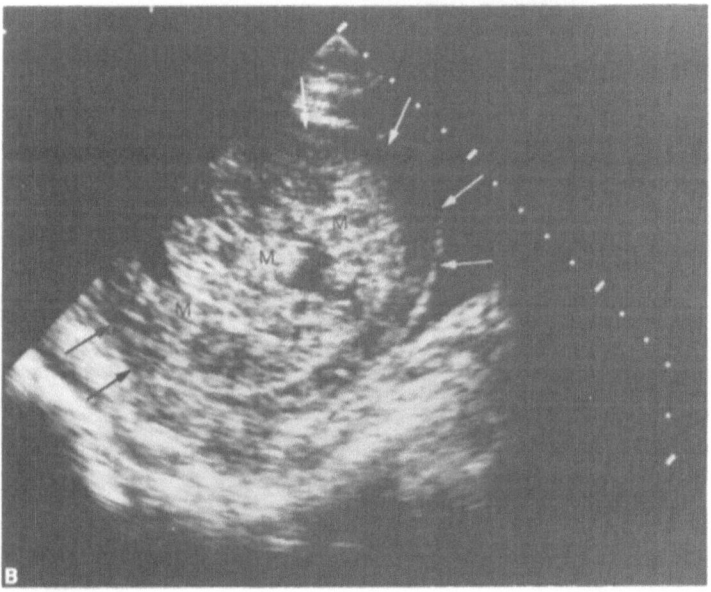

FIG. 15.1.1. MOLAR PREGNANCY

(A) Longitudinal scan demonstrating an enlarged uterus (calipers) with an increase in transonicity (arrows) and echogenicity. No
normal fetal echoes are visualized. Molar tissue (M).

(B) Transverse sector scan demonstrating molar tissue (M) within the uterus (black arrows). Note the absence of normal fetal echoes
and increase in echogenicity. White arrows outline the uterus.

CHAPTER 15 • MOLAR PREGNANCY   **125**

Chapter 16
Second and Third
Trimester Bleeding

16.1. PLACENTA PREVIA (PP)

16.1.1. Low-Lying PP

This condition represents a low-segment placentation. The placenta, however, does not reach the internal os of the cervix (see Fig. 16.1.1A).

16.1.2. Partial PP

The placenta covers part of the internal os of the cervix (see Fig. 16.1.1B).

16.1.3. Complete PP

The placenta fully covers the internal os of the cervix reaching from the anterior to posterior wall of the uterus (see Figs. 16.1.1C and 16.1.2).

- Routine sonography during the second trimester will determine 20% of all pregnancies to have PP. However, the vast majority of these will assume normal positions by term. Only 12% of central PPs discovered during the mid-trimester will remain as such, correcting to a total incidence of 0.5% PPs at term.

- In order to establish the relationship between placenta and internal cervical os, the bladder needs to be filled with approximately 200–250 ml of fluid. It is important to fill the bladder but not to overdistend it; otherwise posterior rotation of the uterus may result, giving the false impression of PP (see Fig. 16.1.3).

- Recognition of a fundal insertion generally precludes the diagnosis of PP.

- Evaluation of a posterior PP is often difficult because of shadowing of fetal parts, particularly the fetal head, when in a vertex presentation.

- The final diagnosis of PP is supported by sonography, but clinical parameters always determine the final diagnosis.

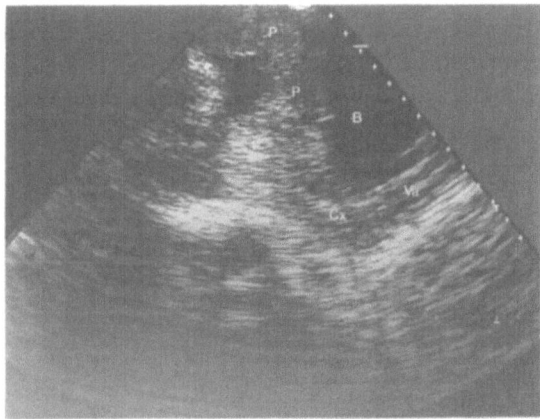

LOW-LYING PLACENTA   PARTIAL PLACENTA PREVIA   TOTAL PLACENTA PREVIA

FIG. 16.1.1. SCHEMATIC REPRESENTATION OF VARIOUS FORMS OF PLACENTA PREVIA

Umbilicus (Um), symphysis pubis (SP), bladder (b), vagina (v), cervix (Cx), placenta (P). (Illustrations by R. V. Giglia.)

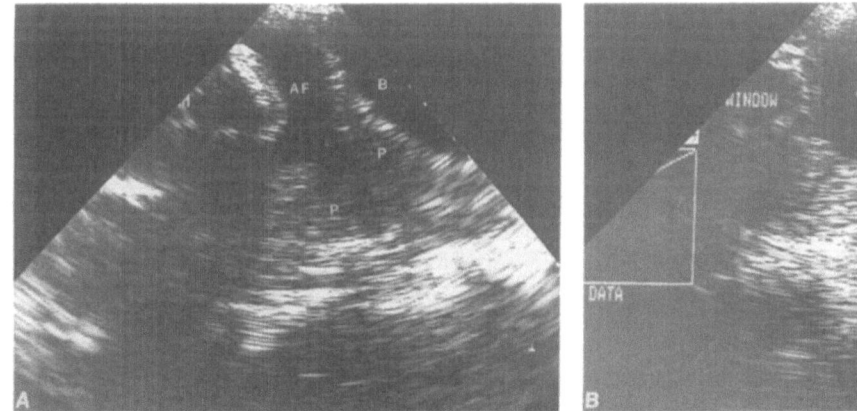

FIG. 16.1.2. SONOGRAPHIC REPRESENTATION OF PLACENTA PREVIA

Longitudinal sector scan demonstrating total placenta previa (P). Bladder (B), cervix (Cx), vagina (Va).

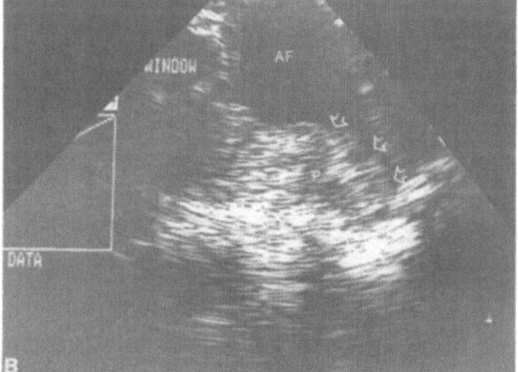

FIG. 16.1.3. POSTVOID EXAMINATION IN SUSPECTED TOTAL PLACENTA PREVIA

Longitudinal sector scans demonstrating the value of the postvoid film when total placenta previa is suspected.

(A)   Total previa when maternal bladder is full. Bladder (B), amniotic fluid (AF), placenta (P).

(B)   Low-lying placenta (open arrows) when the bladder is emptied. Bladder (B), amniotic fluid (AF), placenta (P).

CHAPTER 16 • SECOND AND THIRD TRIMESTER BLEEDING   **129**

16.2. ABRUPTIO PLACENTAE

- The diagnosis of abruptio placentae is a clinical one. Sonography plays only a supportive part.

- Possible sonographic findings (see Fig. 16.2.1) may include the following:

  - A retroplacental echogenic space, which with time may consolidate
  - Extramembraneous fluid collection undergoing similar changes over time

- Abruptions are clinically associated with such conditions as intrauterine growth retardation (IUGR), chronic hypertension. Consequently, sonographic findings typical for those clinical conditions may be associated with abruption:

    Placental calcifications
    Small placental size
    Oligohydramnios

- As part of the differential diagnosis, the following have to be considered:

    Uterine contraction
    Placental cyst
    Myoma uteri
    Maternal venous sinus

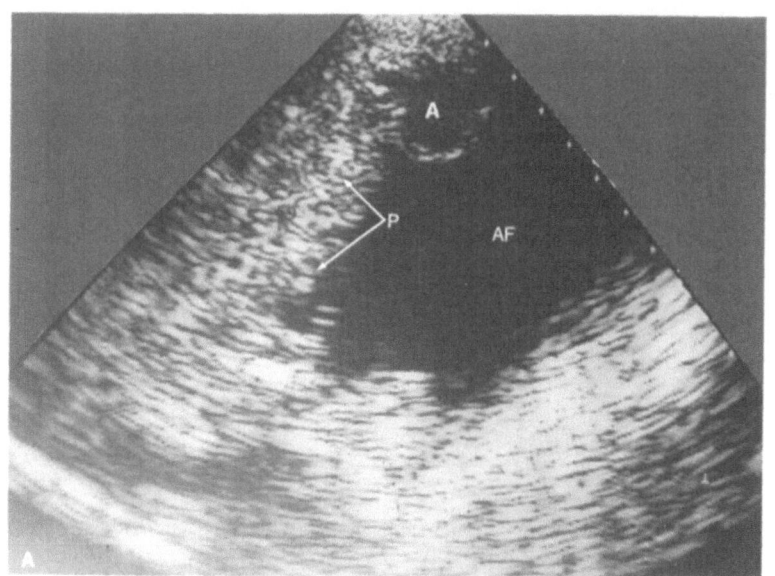

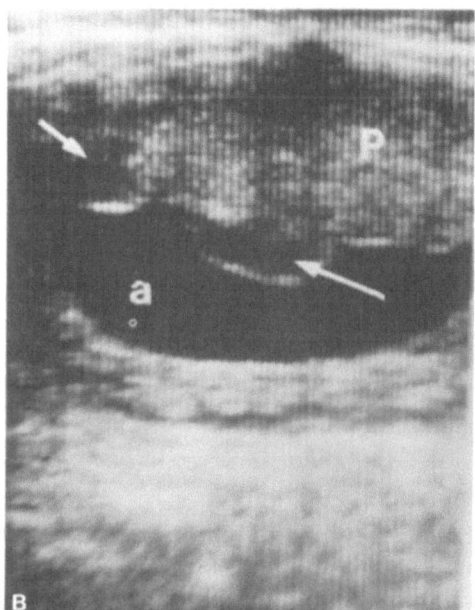

FIG. 16.2.1. PLACENTAL ABRUPTION

(A)   Transverse sector scan demonstrating a clinically suspected abruption (A). Amniotic fluid (AF), placenta (P).

(B)   Echo-spared areas (arrows) within the placenta can be normal findings and can be difficult to distinguish from abruptions. Placenta (P), amniotic fluid (a).

Chapter 17
Abnormal Fetal Anatomy: Level II Sonography

17.1. PRINCIPLES OF LEVEL II SONOGRAPHY:
Target Organ Imaging

- Level II sonography was originally described in the examination of pregnancies characterized by elevated amniotic fluid alpha-fetoprotein. This examination was performed primarily to rule out causes of alpha-fetoprotein elevations (mainly neural tube defects).

- Level II sonography (target organ imaging) in this chapter describes the sonographic examinations of the fetus in an attempt to visualize fetal anomalies (see Table 17.1.1).

- Level II sonography represents a painstakingly detailed and complex sonographic scan that requires both special expertise as well as excessive time (40–60 min) for each patient.

- Current short supply of adequately trained manpower as well as cost-effectiveness considerations preclude routine level II sonography for every patient undergoing obstetric sonography.

- Consequently, only a small group of patients should undergo level II scannings. The following conditions would be included:

  o Maternal diseases resulting in greater frequency of congenital lesions:
    Diabetes mellitus
    Congenital heart disease
  o Clinical suspicion of certain conditions:
    Oligohydramnios
    Polyhydramnios
    Abnormal presentation
    Premature labor
  o Family history of a congenital lesion diagnosable by sonography:
    Congenital renal disease
    Congenital heart disease
  o Genetic diseases diagnosable by sonography:
    Dwarfism
    X-linked aqueductal stenosis
  o Family history of neural tube defects or elevated alpha-fetoprotein levels, or both[1]
  o Suspicious initial scan
  o Fetal hydrops

REFERENCE

1. Hobbins JC, Venus I, Tortora M, et al: Stage II ultrasound examination for the diagnosis of fetal abnormalities with an elevated amniotic fluid alpha-fetoprotein concentration. *Am J Obstet Gynecol* 1982;142:8.

TABLE 17.1.1.

Complete Level II Scan

Sequence of individual steps	To rule out the following lesions
Routine (level I) scan Presentation Number of fetuses and viability Amniotic fluid assessment Placental evaluation Standard biometric parameters	Is performed as an initial scan
Contour of skull	Anencephaly and meningoencephaloceles, cystic hygromas, etc.
Intracranial anatomy of skull	Hydrocephaly, space-occupying lesions
Facial architecture	Cleft lip and palate, epignathus, hypotelorism/hypertelorism
Neck structures	Meningocele and cystic hygroma, thyroid goiter
Vertebral column	Meningomyecocele, sacral agenesis, sacral teratomas
Upper limbs	Skeletal deformities
Thorax	Pleural and pericardial effusions, lung masses and hypoplasia, cardiac defects, diaphragmatic hernias
Abdomen	Hepatobiliary masses, gastrointestinal obstruction
Urinary tract	Urinary tract obstructions, renal agenesis, infantile polycystic kidneys
Genitalia	Congenital hydrocele, sex determination
Lower limbs	Skeletal deformities
Umbilical cord	Single umbilical artery

17.2. THE FETAL HEAD

17.2.1. Disorders Affecting the Continuity of the Skull

- *Anencephaly* represents absence of the cranial vault. Sonographic diagnosis is based on the following findings:

  o   Absence of cranial portion of the skull (see Fig. 17.2.1)
  o   Polyhydramnios in 40% of cases
  o   Prominent facial structures (bulging eyes)

- Additional factors of anencephaly include the following:

  o   Frequently associated with other neural tube defects
  o   Can be reliably diagnosed by 15–16 weeks
  o   Should not be confused with *microcephaly*

- *Encephalocele* represents an ossification defect of the skull.

  o   Can present at any portion of the skull
  o   Frequently associated with *hydrocephaly* and *Meckel's syndrome.*

- *Cystic hygromas* are masses most commonly originating in the neck that result from obstruction of the lymphatic drainage in the neck. Cystic hygromas can also present in the axilla and groin. They may be cystic and very large and contain thick septations when associated with *Turner's (XO) syndrome.* This type of cystic hygroma is almost universally associated with fetal hydrops.[2] Smaller hygromas, with varying echo patterns, have been reported as isolated lesions[2] (see Fig. 17.2.2).

- *Fetal demise* may present sonographically as an overlapping of the skull bones commonly known as *Spalding's sign.*

REFERENCE

2.   Chervenak FA, Isaacson G, Blakemore KJ, et al: Fetal cystic hygroma: Cause and natural history. *N Engl J Med* 1983;309:822.

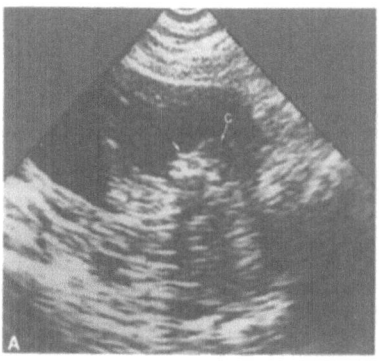 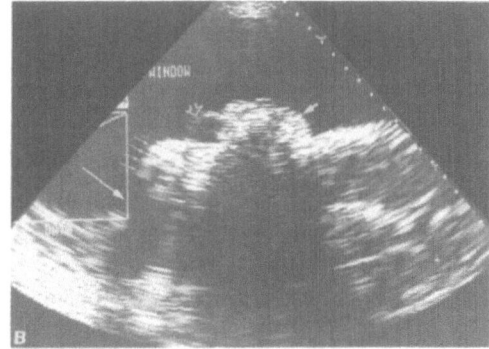

FIG. 17.2.1. ANENCEPHALY AND ENCEPHALOCELE

(A) Transverse sector scan demonstrating an anencephalic fetus at 13 weeks gestation. Note the prominent facial bones (small arrow) and absence of the cranial vault (C). Caution is recommended when making a diagnosis of early anencephaly because of possible confusion over incorrect dates and possible microcephaly. Reliable confirmation is possible by 15–16 weeks gestation.

(B) Longitudinal sector scan through the fetal cranium demonstrating the mandible (single arrow), orbit (open arrow), and a portion of the frontal bones (small arrows). This case shows no evidence of a cranial vault, suggesting anencephaly.

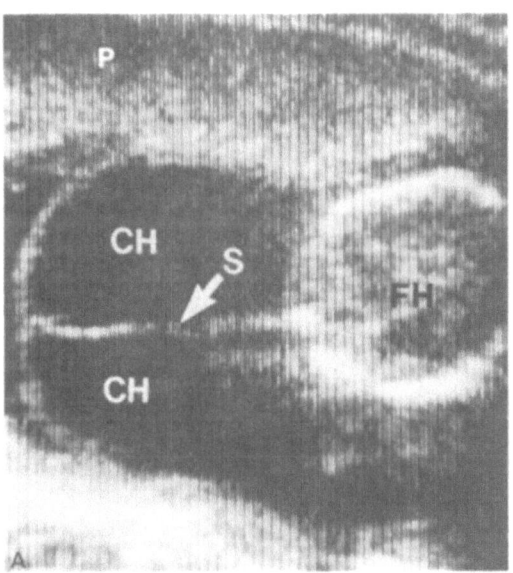 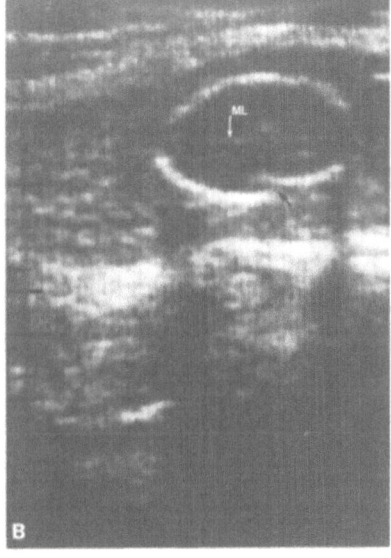

FIG. 17.2.2. FETUS WITH TURNER'S SYNDROME

(A) Transverse scan through the fetal head (FH) demonstrating a large *cystic hygroma* (CH). Note the midline septum (S). Placenta (P).
From Chervenak et al.[2]

(B) Transverse scan through the fetal skull demonstrating overlapping of the skull bones (arrow), indicating *Spalding's sign*, commonly seen with a fetal demise. Midline (ML).

17.2.2. Intracranial Anatomy

- *Hydrocephaly* is the abnormal dilatation of the lateral ventricles (see Figs. 17.2.3 and 17.2.4).

    o With modern obstetric sonography, biparietal diameter (BPD) measurements cannot be relied on to make the diagnosis of hydrocephaly.[3]

    o Direct ventricular diameter measurements permit the diagnosis of early hydrocephaly.

    o The diagnostic assessment of ventricular diameter can be made by the use of nomograms (see Table 17.2.1).[4] This technique is described in Section 4.2.

    o The lateral ventricular/hemispheric width ratio[4] can be used to calculate the degree of ventricular dilation (see Section 4.2.).

TABLE 17.2.1
Calculated Values from Regression Equation of Bifrontal Horn Width

BPD (cm)	Mean (cm)	Vetricular ratio	Upper 95% CL (cm)	Upper 99% CL (cm)	BPD (cin)	Mean (cm)	Ventricular ratio	Upper 95% CL (cm)	Upper 99% CL (cm)
2.3	1.1	0.48	1.36	1.45	6.2	1.8	0.28	2.01	2.09
2.4	1.1	0.47	1.39	1.48	6.3	1.8	0.28	2.03	2.10
2.5	1.2	0.47	1.42	1.51	6.4	1.8	0.28	2.04	2.12
2.6	1.2	0.46	1.46	1.54	6.5	1.8	0.28	2.06	2.14
2.7	1.2	0.46	1.48	1.56	6.6	1.8	0.28	2.08	2.15
2.8	1.3	0.45	1.51	1.59	6.7	1.8	0.28	2.09	2.17
2.9	1.3	0.45	1.54	1.62	6.8	1.9	0.27	2.11	2.19
3.0	1.3	0.44	1.57	1.65	6.9	1.9	0.27	2.13	2.21
3.1	1.3	0.43	1.59	1.67	7.0	1.9	0.27	2.15	2.23
3.2	1.4	0.43	1.61	1.69	7.1	1.9	0.27	2.17	2.25
3.3	1.4	0.42	1.63	1.71	7.2	1.9	0.27	2.19	2.27
3.4	1.4	0.41	1.65	1.73	7.3	2.0	0.27	2.21	2.29
3.5	1.4	0.41	1.67	1.75	7.4	2.0	0.27	2.24	2.31
3.6	1.4	0.40	1.69	1.77	7.5	2.0	0.27	2.26	2.35
3.7	1.5	0.39	1.70	1.78	7.6	2.0	0.27	2.28	2.36
3.8	1.5	0.39	1.72	1.80	7.7	2.1	0.27	2.30	2.38
3.9	1.5	0.38	1.73	1.81	7.8	2.1	0.27	2.33	2.40
4.0	1.5	0.37	1.74	1.82	7.9	2.1	0.27	2.34	2.43
4.1	1.5	0.37	1.76	1.84	8.0	2.1	0.27	2.37	2.45
4.2	1.5	0.36	1.77	1.85	8.1	2.1	0.27	2.39	2.47
4.3	1.5	0.36	1.78	1.86	8.2	2.2	0.26	2.42	2.50
4.4	1.5	0.35	1.79	1.87	8.3	2.2	0.26	2.44	2.52
4.5	1.6	0.35	1.80	1.88	8.4	2.2	0.26	2.46	2.54
4.6	1.6	0.34	1.81	1.89	8.5	2.2	0.26	2.49	2.57
4.7	1.6	0.34	1.82	1.90	8.6	2.3	0.26	2.51	2.59
4.8	1.6	0.33	1.83	1.91	8.7	2.3	0.26	2.53	2.61
4.9	1.6	0.33	1.84	1.92	8.8	2.3	0.26	2.55	2.63
5.0	1.6	0.32	1.85	1.93	8.9	2.3	0.26	2.57	2.65
5.1	1.6	0.32	1.87	1.95	9.0	2.3	0.26	2.59	2.67
5.2	1.6	0.31	1.88	1.96	9.1	2.4	0.26	2.61	2.69
5.3	1.6	0.31	1.89	1.97	9.2	2.4	0.26	2.63	2.71
5.4	1.7	0.31	1.90	1.98	9.3	2.4	0.26	2.65	2.73
5.5	1.7	0.30	1.91	1.99	9.4	2.4	0.26	2.67	2.75
5.6	1.7	0.30	1.92	2.00	9.5	2.4	0.26	2.69	2.77
5.7	1.7	0.30	1.94	2.02	9.6	2.4	0.25	2.70	2.78
5.8	1.7	0.29	1.95	2.03	9.7	2.5	0.25	2.72	2.80
5.9	1.7	0.29	1.96	2.04	9.8	2.5	0.25	2.74	2.82
6.0	1.7	0.29	1.98	2.06	9.9	2.5	0.25	2.77	2.85
6.1	1.7	0.29	1.99	2.07	10.0	2.5	0.25	2.79	2.87

From Denkhaus and Winsberg.[4]

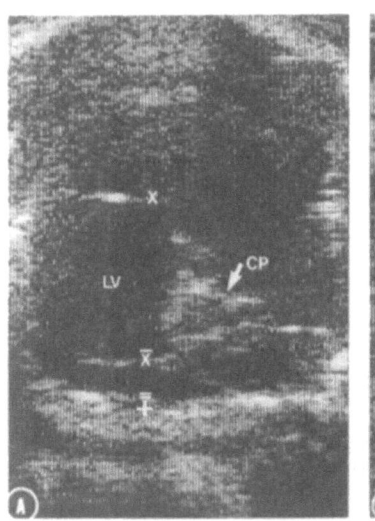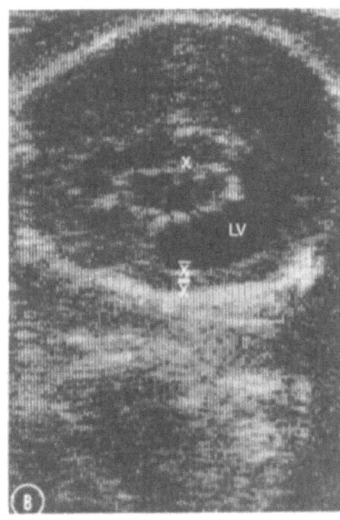

FIG. 17.2.3. MACROCEPHALY AND MICROCEPHALY IN CONJUNCTION WITH HYDROCEPHALUS

(A) Transverse scan through the fetal head demonstrating macrocephaly (BPD 93 mm at 33 weeks Gestation) and hydrocephalus. Dilated lateral ventricle (LV), choroid plexus (CP), midline echo (X), lateral wall of lateral ventricle (X̌), inner skull table (X). The lateral ventricle:hemispheric width ratio was 77%.

(B) Transverse scan demonstrating microcephaly (BPD 62 mm at 33 weeks gestation) and hydrocephaly. Dilated ventricle (LV), midline echo (X), lateral wall of lateral ventricle (X̌), inner skull table (X̿).
From Chervenak et al.[3]

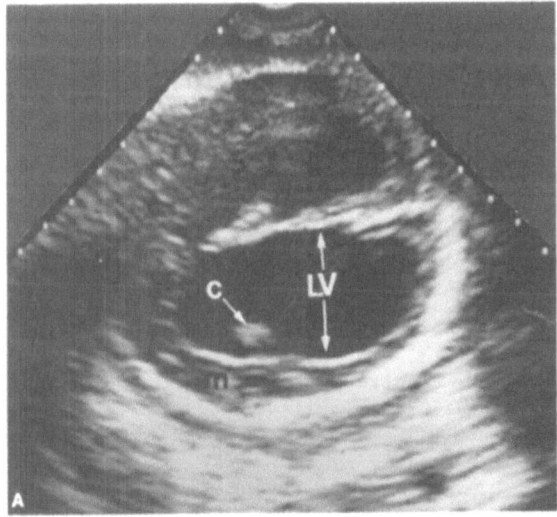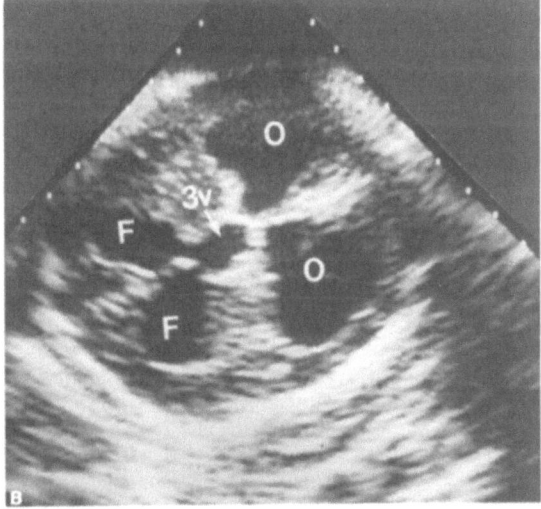

FIG. 17.2.4. HYDROCEPHALUS AT 27 WEEKS AT DIFFERENT SCANNING LEVELS

(A) Transverse sector scan at the level of the lateral ventricles demonstrating hydrocephalus at 27 weeks gestation. Dilated lateral ventricle (LV), choroid plexus (c), and cortical mantle (m).

(B) Transverse sector scan at the level of the third ventricle (3v) in the same patient demonstrating dilated frontal (F) and occipital (O) horns. Note the dilated third ventricle.
From Grannum et al.[6]

- o Hydrocephalus is highly associated with other major congenital abnormalities. A recent study showed only 15% of cases to involve an isolated hydrocephalus.[3]
- o When hydrocephaly is believed to represent an isolated lesion, is diagnosed early, and when brain tissue is still appreciable, intrauterine shunting under sonographic control has been successfully achieved.[5]

REFERENCES

3. Chervenak FA, Berkowitz RL, Romero R, et al: The diagnosis of fetal hydrocephalus. *Am J Obstet Gynecol* 1983;147:703.
4. Denkhaus H, Winsberg F: Ultrasonic measurement of the fetal ventricular system. *Radiology* 1979;131:781.
5. Clewell WH, Johnson ML, Meier PR, et al: A surgical approach to the treatment of fetal hydrocephalus. *N Engl J Med* 1982;306:1320.
6. Grannum PAT, Tortora M, Mayden KL, Taylor KJW: Obstetrical ultrasound, in Taylor KJW (ed): *Atlas of Ultrasonography,* ed 2. New York, Churchill Livingstone, 1985.

17.2.3. The Face

- In many genetic syndromes subtle defects of the face may occur in conjunction with major cranial abnormalities.

- *Cleft lip and palate* represents a difficult sonographic diagnosis. Nevertheless, cases of sonographically diagnosed cleft lip and palate have been reported[7,8] (see Fig. 17.2.5).

- *Hypotelorism and hypertelorism* represent abnormally spaced orbits. These conditions are commonly found in association with other cranial abnormalities[9] (see Figs. 17.2.5 and 17.2.6).

- *Masses of the oral cavity* may represent a rare condition such as teratoma.

REFERENCES

7. Chervenak FA, Tortora M, Mayden KL, et al: Median cleft face syndrome: Antenatal sonographic demonstration of cleft lip and hypertelorism. *Am J Obstet Gynecol* 1984;149:94.
8. Christ JE, Meniger MG: Ultrasonic diagnosis of cleft lip and cleft palate before birth. *Reconstr Surg* 1981;6:854.
9. Mayden KL, Tortora M, Berkowitz RL, et al: Orbital diameters: A new parameter for prenatal diagnosis and dating. *Am J Obstet Gynecol* 1982;144:289.
10. Chervenak FA, Isaacson G, Mahoney MJ, et al: The obstetrical significance of holoprosencephaly. *Obstet Gynecol* 1984;63:115.

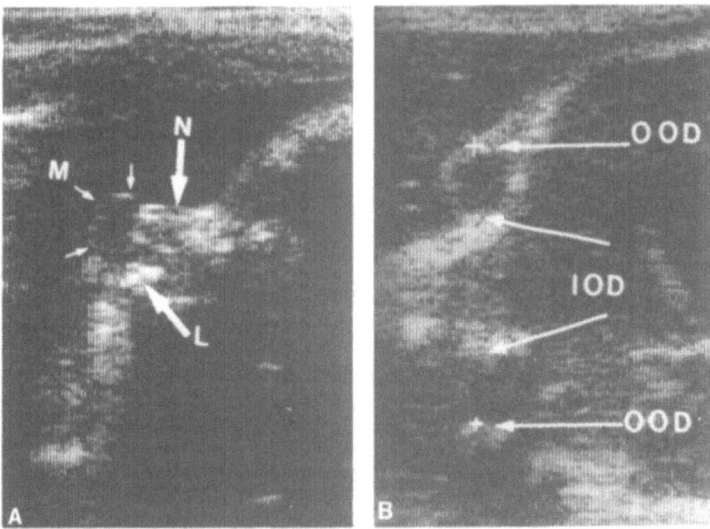

FIG. 17.2.5. CLEFT LIP AND HYPERTELORISM IN A 31-WEEK FETUS (MEDIAN CLEFT FACE SYNDROME)

(A) Profile of the fetal face depicting the nose (N) and a protruding soft tissue mass (M). Lip (L).

(B) Transverse sonogram demonstrating the outer orbital distance (OOD) and the inner orbital distance (IOD) at 31 weeks gestation. Both orbital distances were above the 95% confidence limits, suggesting hypertelorism.
From Chervenak et al.[7]

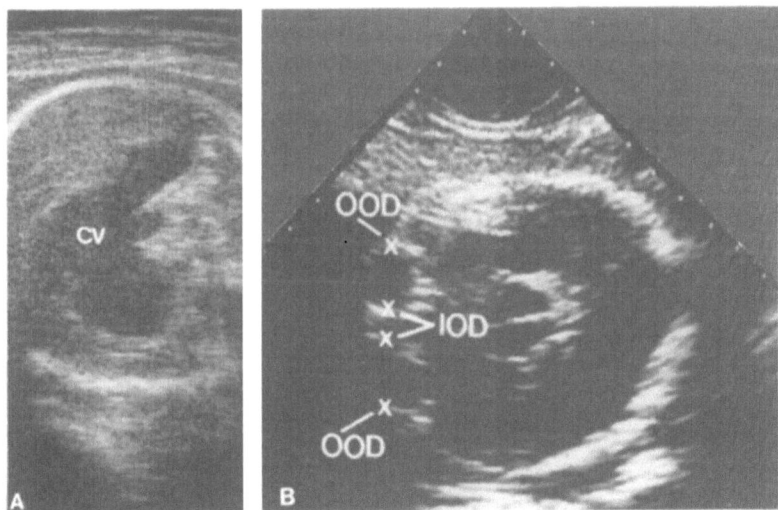

FIG. 17.2.6. HYPOTELORISM IN ASSOCIATION WITH HOLOPROSENCEPHALY AT 28 WEEKS

(A) Transverse scan through the fetal head at 28 weeks gestation demonstrating a common ventricle (CV). Note the absence of the central midline.

(B) Transverse sector scan demonstrating the outer orbital distance (OOD) and inner orbital distance (IOD) in the same fetus with holoprosencephaly. Orbital distances were below the 95% confidence limits, suggesting hypotelorism.
From Chervenak et al.[10]

17.2.4. The Spine

The routine scanning process of the fetal spine is described in Section 4.3. Abnormalities that may be sonographically detected are the following:

- *Spina bifida (cystica)* represents incomplete closure of the neural tube, resulting in protrusion of meninges and frequently of the spinal cord (see Fig. 17.2.7).

  - o During the scanning process, every vertebra needs to be evaluated.
  - o Despite such detailed efforts, many small neural tube defects will not be diagnosed.
  - o This condition is highly associated with hydrocephaly.

- *Sacrococcygeal teratoma* represents a cystic–solid tumor arising from the sacrum (see Fig. 17.2.8).

  - o Needs to be differentiated from a low meningomyelocele

- *Sacral agenesis* is reported as increased in the offspring of diabetic pregnancies.

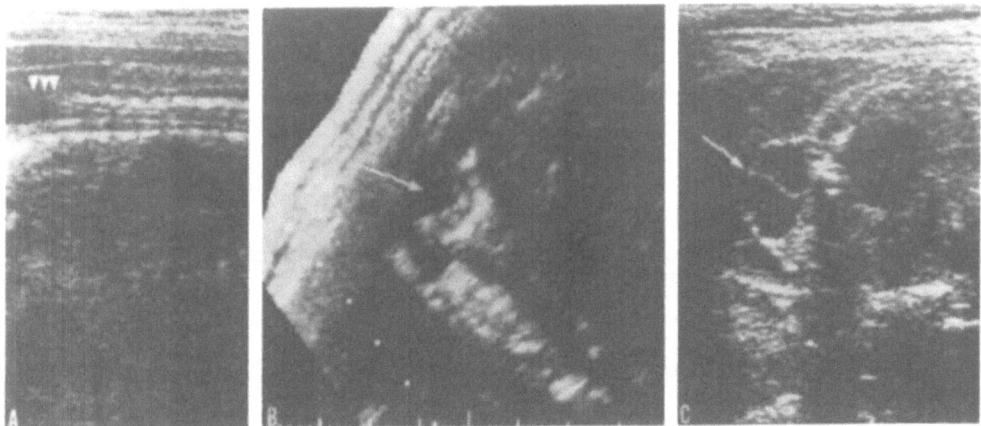

FIG. 17.2.7. OPEN SPINAL DEFECTS

(A) Longitudinal scan demonstrating open spinal defect (arrows).

(B) Transverse scan of same patient, demonstrating spinal defect (arrow).

(C) Transverse scan demonstrating meningomyelocele with covering membrane (arrow).
From Chervenak *et al.*[3]

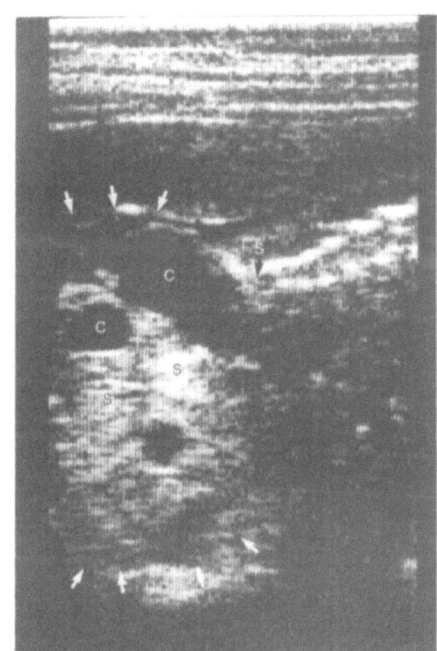

FIG. 17.2.8. SACROCOCCYGEAL TERATOMA

Longitudinal scan demonstrating the sacrum (S) with a coexisting complex mass
(arrows). Note both the cystic (C) and solid black (S) components.
From Grannum *et al.*[6]

17.3. UPPER LIMBS

- In skeletal dysplasias sonography may be diagnostic in demonstrating either a reduction in long bone length, evidence of bone fractures, or a decrease in bone density (hypomineralization).[11,12]

- Deformities of the fetal hand may include the following sonographic diagnoses:

  - Polydactyly (i.e., Ellis-Van Crevald syndrome)
  - Syndactyly
  - Lobster claw deformity

- Deformities of the long bones may include the following sonographic diagnoses:

  - Osteogenesis imperfecta (see Fig. 17.3.1)
  - Achondroplasia
  - Thanatophoric dysplasia (see Fig. 17.7.1)

REFERENCES

11. Chervenak FA, Romero RR, Berkowitz RL, et al: Antenatal sonographic findings of osteogenesis imperfecta. *Am J Obstet Gynecol* 1982;143:288.
12. Grannum PAT, Hobbins JC: Prenatal diagnosis of fetal skeletal dysplasias. *Semin Perinatol* 1983;7:125.

17.4. THE FETAL THORAX

17.4.1. The Fetal Ribs

With certain skeletal dysplasias such as *osteogenesis imperfecta,* rib fractures potentially may be found sonographically.

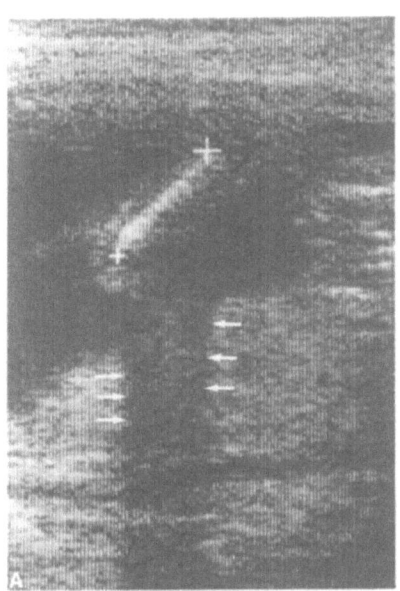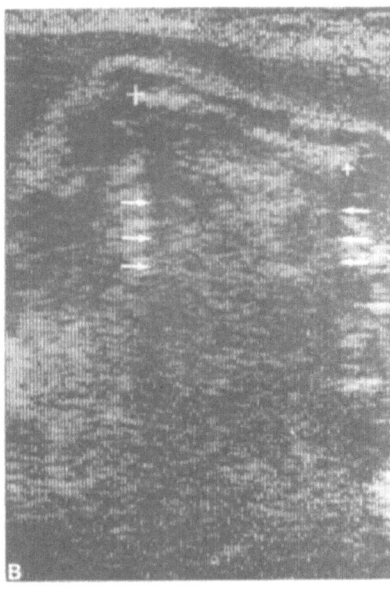

FIG. 17.3.1. OSTEOGENESIS IMPERFECTA AT 24 WEEKS

(A) Longitudinal scan depicting the humeral length (calipers) at 20 weeks gestation. The humeral length was below the 95% confidence limit and osteogenesis imperfecta was suspected. No obvious fractures were noted. Note the acoustic shadowing (arrows) from the humerus.

(B) Longitudinal scan of the humerus in the same patient at 24 weeks gestation. The humeral length remained below the 95% confidence limit. Note the decrease in acoustic shadowing from the humerus (arrows).
From Chervenak *et al.*[11]

17.4.2. The Fetal Lungs and Diaphragm

Lung masses can be visualized antenatally and need to be differentiated from diaphragmatic hernias, cardiac abnormalities, and pleural effusions[13] (see Fig. 17.4.1):

- *Simple lung cysts* represents clear cystic spaces within the lung parenchyma.

- *Solid lung masses* may include the following sonographic findings:
    - Adenomatoid malformations
    - Pulmonary sequestrations

- *Complex lung masses* (represented as either cystic or solid or a combination of cystic/solid components) may include several findings:
    - Cystic dilation of the bronchus
    - Adenomatoid malformations
    - Encephaloceles
    - Pulmonary sequestrations

- *Diaphragmatic hernia*[14] represents the absence of a part of the diaphragm and intrusion of abdominal contents into the chest cavity. The sonographic diagnosis is made by demonstrating the following:
    - Fetal bowel, stomach, or liver in the chest cavity (see Fig. 17.4.2)
    - Hypoplasia of the lung

- *Pleural effusion* is rarely an isolated lesion. This condition is usually associated with other signs of immunologic or nonimmunologic hydrops (see Chapters 10 and 11 and Fig. 17.4.3).

REFERENCES

13. Mayden KL, Tortora M, Chervenak FA, et al: The antenatal sonographic detection of lung masses. *Am J Obstet Gynecol* 1984;148:3.
14. Hobbins JC, Grannum PAT, Berkowitz RL, et al: Ultrasound in the diagnosis of congenital anomalies. *Am J Obstet Gynecol* 1979;134:331.

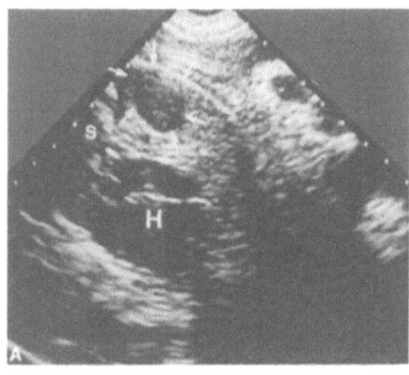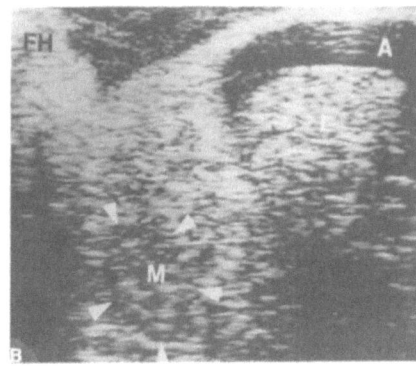

FIG. 17.4.1. FETAL LUNG MASSES

(A) Transverse sector scan demonstrating an echo-spared mass (arrows) in the lung. Note the relationship of this mass to the fetal heart (H). This mass was consistent with a congenital bronchial cyst. Spine (S).

(B) Longitudinal scan through the fetal upper abdomen demonstrating an echo-dense lung mass (M, arrows). Fetal ascites (A) was noted. Liver (L), fetal head (FH). Postmortem examination revealed an adenomatoid malformation. From Mayden et al.[13]

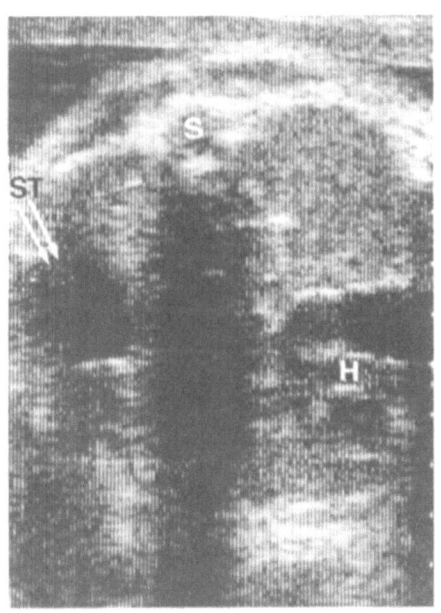

FIG. 17.4.2. DIAPHRAGMATIC HERNIA

Transverse scan of the fetal thorax with the fetus in a spine-up (S) position. The fetal stomach (ST) is noted at the same level as the fetal heart (H), which is indicative of a diaphragmatic hernia. (Courtesy of the Perinatal Ultrasound Unit, Yale New Haven Medical Center, New Haven, Connecticut.)

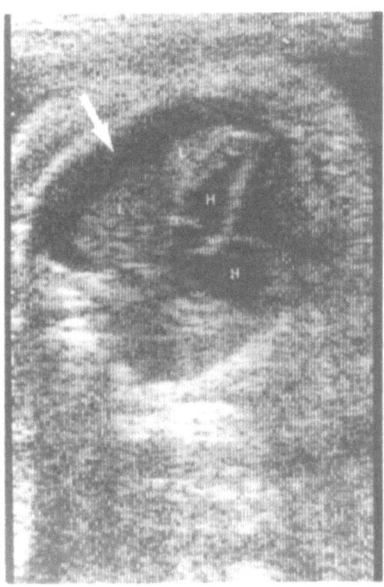

FIG. 17.4.3. PLEURAL EFFUSION WITH PULMONARY HYPOPLASIA

Transverse scan demonstrating a pleural effusion (arrow). The fetal lung (L) and heart (H) are also visualized. From Grannum et al.[6]

17.4.3. The Fetal Heart

The fetal heart can be evaluated sonographically in two aspects: first for *rhythm disorders* and second for *structural disorders*[15]:

- *Rhythm disorders* include the following sonographic diagnoses:

  o Supraventricular tachyarrhythmia
  o Complete (third-degree) atrioventricular block

- *Structural disorders* that are most frequently diagnosed sonographically include the following:

  o Septal defects (see Fig. 17.4.4)
  o Single ventricle
  o Hypoplastic left heart
  o Congenital rhabdomyosarcoma of the heart

- *Pericardial effusions* usually only occur in conjunction with immunologic or nonimmunologic hydrops (see Chapters 10 and 11).

- M-mode echocardiography is widely used in the prenatal diagnosis of congenital heart disease.

- Once a major congenital cardiac anomaly has been established sonographically, a complete level II scan is indicated because of the extremely high incidence of major associated abnormalities.

REFERENCES

15. Kleinman CS, Donnerstein RL, DeVore GR, et al: Fetal echocardiography for evaluation of in utero congestive heart failure: A technique for study of non-immune fetal hydrops. *N Engl J Med* 1982;306:568.

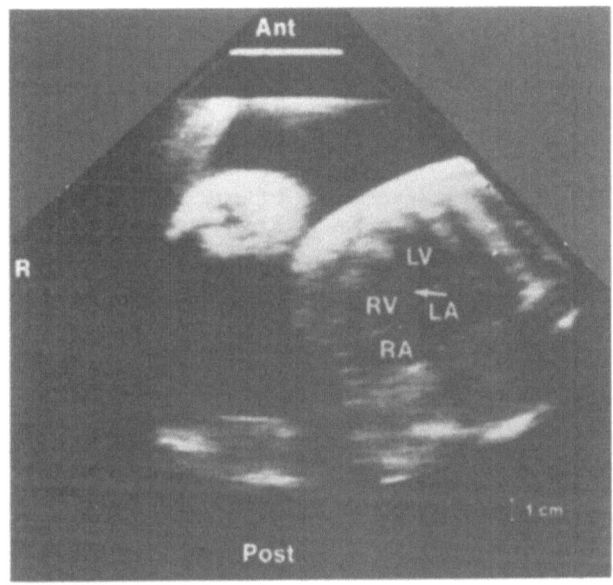

FIG. 17.4.4. INTRAVENTRICULAR SEPTAL DEFECT

A large interventricular septal defect (arrow) is evident in this four-chamber view. The inlet septum and interatrial septum are deficient of tissue and should have suggested the diagnosis of atrioventricular-canal defect. Left atrium (LA), right atrium (RA), left ventricle (LV), right atrium (RA).
From Kleinman *et al.*[15]

17.5. THE FETAL ABDOMEN

17.5.1. Abdominal Wall Defects

- *Omphalocele*: Represents the failure of abdominal contents to return to the abdominal cavity. Abdominal contents are thus sonographically visible within a dilated umbilical sac into which the umbilical cord enters. This lesion is highly associated with chromosomal and multiple congenital abnormalities (see Fig. 17.5.1).

- *Gastroschisis*: Represents a primary abdominal wall defect with free-floating eviscerated abdominal organs. The cord insertion, however, is usually to the right of the lesion and is normal (see Fig. 17.5.2).

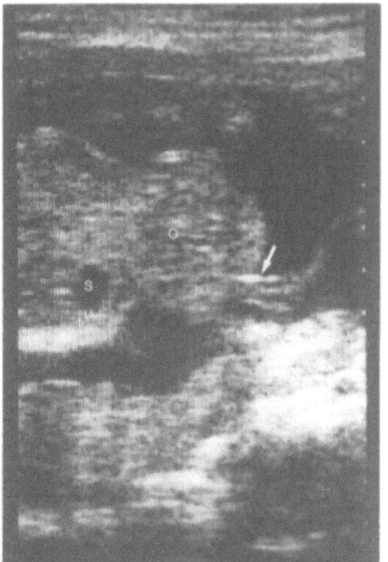

FIG. 17.5.1. OMPHALOCELE

Transverse scan of the fetal abdomen at the level of the umbilicus demonstrating an omphalocele (O) and entrance of the cord into the omphalocele (arrow). The fetal stomach (S) is noted at the peripheral border of the abdomen.
(Courtesy of the Perinatal Ultrasound Unit, Yale New Haven Medical Center, New Haven, Connecticut.)

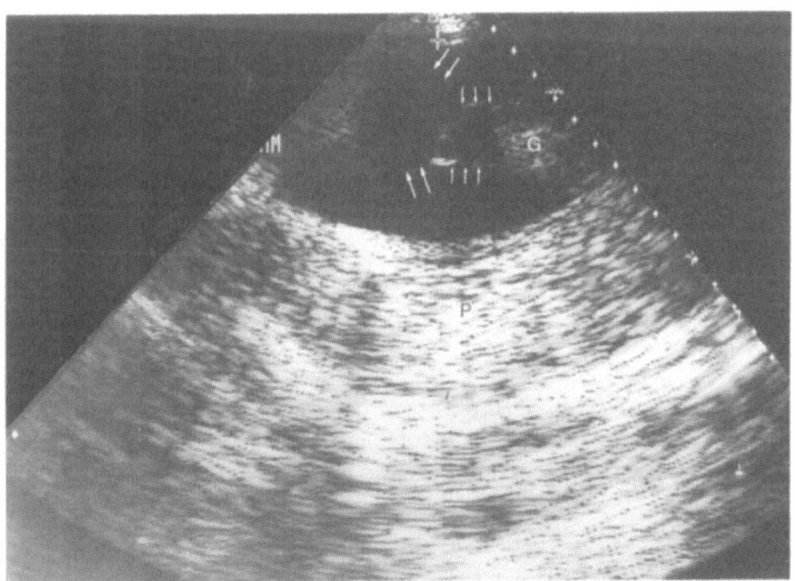

FIG. 17.5.2. GASTROSCHISIS

Oblique sector scan demonstrating bands (arrows) coming from the protruding abdominal contents (G), which was associated with a gastroschisis. Placenta (P).

17.5.2. Gastrointestinal Defects

- *Esophageal atresia* can be suspected with polyhydramnios and repeated absence of a gastric bubble. The definitive sonographic diagnosis is, however, difficult.

- *Duodenal atresia* can be sonographically diagnosed by demonstration of the classic *double bubble sign*. Because of its association with chromosomal and associated abnormalities, level II sonography is indicated (see Figs. 17.5.3 and 17.5.4).

- *Intestinal obstruction* is sonographically similar to the findings in the adult; large bowel loops, representing sonographically large cystic spaces, can be observed. Obstruction may be caused by several conditions:
  - Meconium ileus
  - Volvulus
  - Cystic fibrosis
  - Anal atresia
  - Congenital microcolon

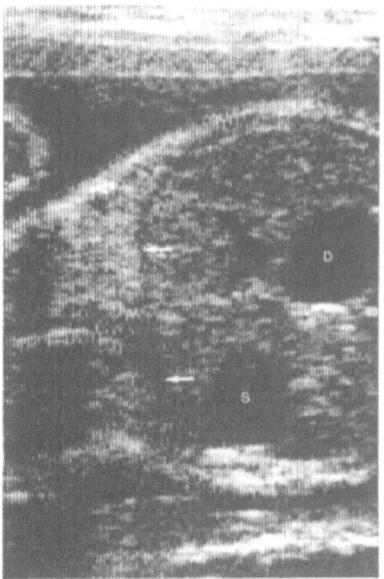

FIG. 17.5.3. DUODENAL ATRESIA

Longitudinal scan demonstrating the typical double-bubble appearance of duodenal atresia located below the fetal diaphragm (arrow). Stomach (S), duodenum (D). From Grannum et al.[6]

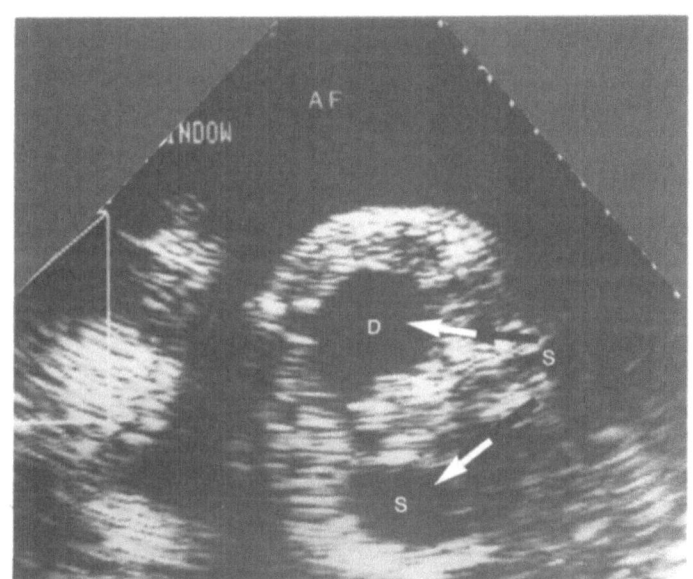

FIG. 17.5.4. DUODENAL ATRESIA

Transverse sector scan depicting the double-bubble sign (white arrows) typical of duodenal atresia. The dilated stomach (S) and duodenum (D) can be identified. Amniotic fluid (AF).

17.5.3. Hepatobiliary System Defects

The following lesions have been sonographically diagnosed:

- Hepatic cysts
- Choledochal cysts (see Fig. 17.5.5)
- Pancreatic cysts

17.5.4. Abdominal Cysts

- Omental cysts
- Ovarian cysts
- Intra-abdominal tumors

REFERENCES

16. Elrad H, Mayden KL, Gleicher N, et al: Prenatal diagnosis of choledochal cyst. *J Ultrasound Med* 1985;4:553–555.

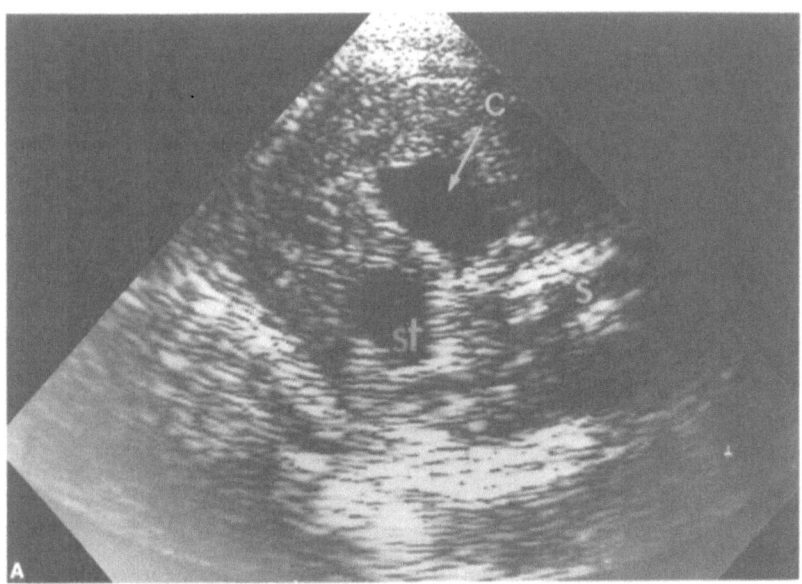

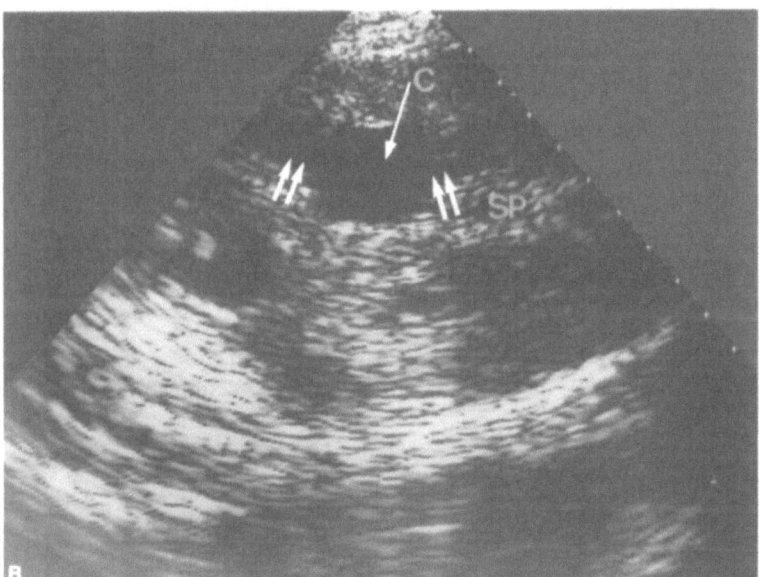

FIG. 17.5.5. CHOLEDOCHAL CYST AT 29 WEEKS GESTATIONAL AGE

(A) Transverse sector scan demonstrating an echo-spared mass (C) in the right upper quadrant. The fetal stomach (st) can be identified to the left of the cyst. Spine (S).

(B) Transverse sector scan demonstrating the echo-spared mass (C) in the same patient. Tubular structures were noted at both ends of the mass (arrows). Spine (SP).
From Elrad *et al.*[16]

17.6. THE URINARY TRACT

17.6.1. The Fetal Kidney

The fetal kidney may show the following abnormalities:

- *Congenital absence (renal agenesis)* (see Fig. 17.6.1). The sonographic diagnosis is based on the following:

  - Severe oligohydramnios
  - Nonvisualization of the bladder, even after furosemide (lasix) challenge
  - Because adrenals may mimic the absent kidneys, the diagnosis may be difficult.

- *Polycystic (infantile) kidneys* (see Fig. 17.6.2) is sonographically defined by the following:

  - Severe oligohydramnios
  - Nonvisualization of the bladder
  - Enlarged, echo-dense kidneys with a central echo-free area
  - Total kidney circumference larger than one-third of the abdominal circumference (see also Section 4.8)

- *Multicystic kidneys* represent large cystic kidneys that may be either unilateral or bilateral; they are sonographically characterized by cysts of varying sizes.

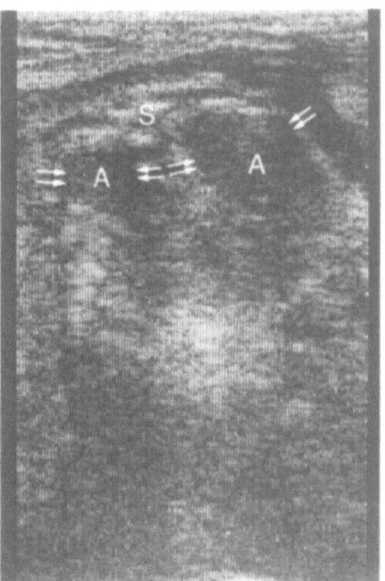

FIG. 17.6.1. RENAL AGENESIS

Transverse scan through the lower fetal abdomen demonstrating enlarged fetal adrenals (A) with the fetus in a spine-up (S) position. Note the absence of normal renal characteristics.

(Courtesy of the Perinatal Ultrasound Unit, Yale New Haven Medical Center, New Haven, Connecticut.)

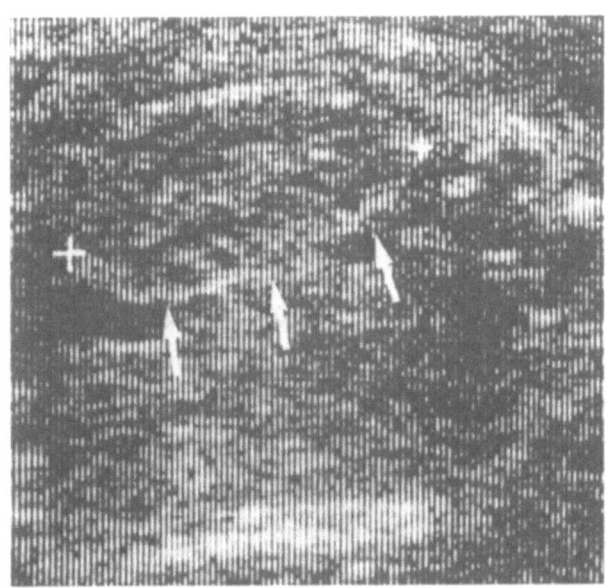

FIG. 17.6.2. INFANTILE POLYCYSTIC KIDNEYS

Transverse scan through the fetal abdomen demonstrating an enlarged echo-dense kidney (arrows) consistent with a polysystic kidney. From Chervenak et al.[3]

17.6.2. Urinary Tract Obstruction

- *Ureteral obstruction* may occur at different levels; it may be unilateral or bilateral and complete or incomplete. The most frequent sites of obstruction are the following:

    o Ureteropelvic junction (UPJ) (see Fig. 17.6.3)
    o Ureterovesical junction (UVJ)

    The sonographic picture will be dependent on site, uni- or bilaterality, and complete or incomplete obstruction. With *complete bilateral* obstruction, the sonographic picture will be that of several findings:

    o Oligohydramnios
    o Nonvisualization of bladder
    o Ureteral dilatation
    o Enlargement of kidneys (hydronephrosis)
    o Occasional fetal ascites

    With *incomplete or unilateral obstruction,* there are only two signs:

    o Ureteral dilatation
    o Hydronephrotic kidneys (see Fig. 17.6.4)

    Urinary diversion *in utero* has recently been suggested by some investigators.[17,18] Diversion appears to be a consideration only if the diagnosis is made early, obstruction is bilateral, and renal parenchyma is considered salvageable. This is an experimental procedure.

- *Urethra and bladder.* Obstruction of the urethra is usually caused by a *posterior uretheral valve* (PUV) (see Fig. 17.6.5). The sonographic picture includes the following:

    o Frequent oligohydramnios (see Fig. 17.6.6)
    o Enlarged bladder
    o Hydroureters
    o Hydronephrosis
    o Visible urethra
    o Occasional visible urethra

    PUV represents an intermittent obstruction; surgical considerations *in utero* are similar to those noted above.

REFERENCES

17. Golbus MS, Harrison MR, Filly RA, et al: In utero treatment of urinary tract obstruction. *Am J Obstet Gynecol* 1982;142:383.
18. Berkowitz RL, Glickman MG, Smith GJW, et al: Fetal urinary tract obstruction: What is the role of surgical intervention in utero? *Am J Obstet Gynecol* 1982;144:367.

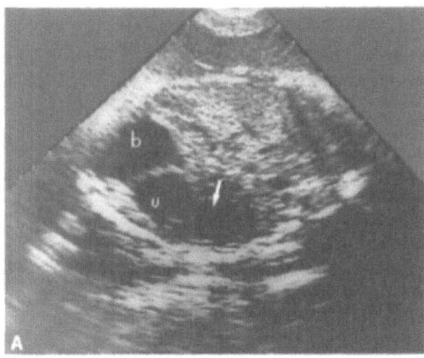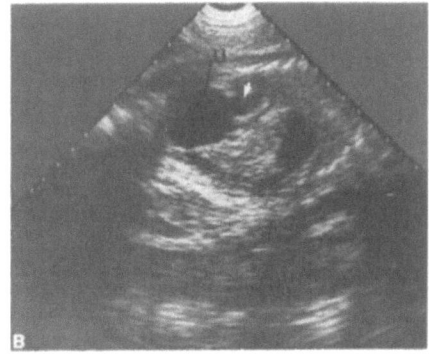

FIG. 17.6.3. UNILATERAL URETERAL OBSTRUCTION (A) Sagittal sector scan through the lower fetal abdomen at 26 weeks gestation demonstrating a dilated renal pelvis (large arrow), and ureter (u). The bladder (b) was identified and of normal size. (B) Oblique sector scan in the same patient depicting the dilated ureter (u) entering the renal pelvis (small white arrow).

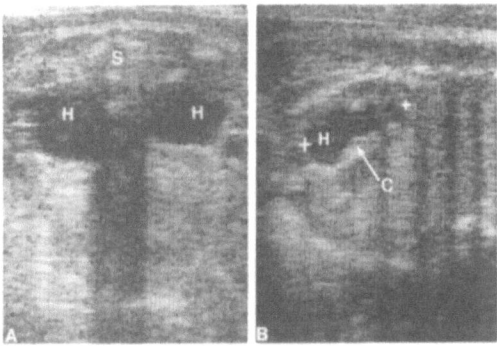

FIG. 17.6.4. HYDRONEPHROSIS (A) Transverse scan through the fetal abdomen demonstrating hydronephrosis (H) bilaterally. Spine (S). (B) Longitudinal scan of same patient demonstrating the dilated renal pelvis (H) and renal cortex (C). From Grannum et al.[6]

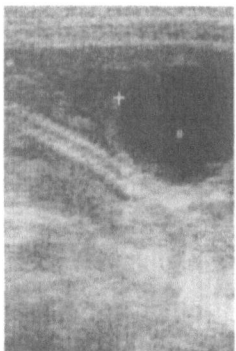

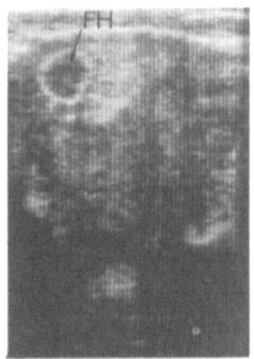

FIG. 17.6.5. POSTERIOR URETHRAL VALVE SYNDROME Longitudinal scan demonstrating an enlarged bladder (B) at 16 weeks gestation. Spine (S). From Grannum et al.[6]

FIG. 17.6.6. OLIGOHYDRAMNIOS WITH URINARY TRACT OBSTRUCTION Transverse scan of an 18-week gestation demonstrating severe oligohydramnios in a fetus with urinary obstruction. Fetal head (FH).

17.7. LOWER LIMBS

17.7.1. Skeletal Dysplasias

Lower limb bones may play the same sonographic part as upper limb bones (see Section 17.3). (See Fig. 17.7.1.)

17.7.2. Clubfoot

Clubfoot has been sonographically diagnosed[19] (see Fig. 17.7.2).

REFERENCE

19. Chervenak FA, Tortora M, Hobbins JC: Antenatal sonographic diagnosis of clubfoot. *J Ultrasound Med* 1985;4:49.

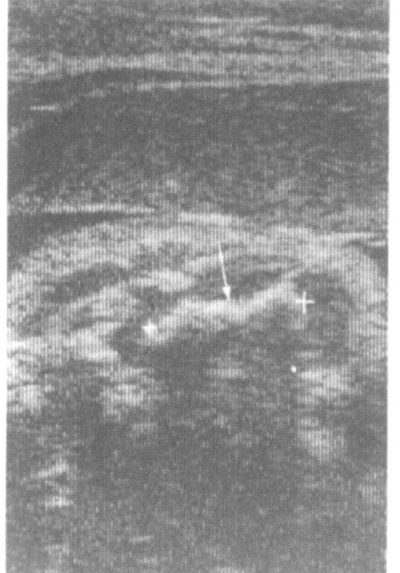

FIG. 17.7.1. THANATOPHORIC DYSPLASIA

Longitudinal scan demonstrating a femur (arrow and calipers) that is markedly short-ened for the gestational age (below 95th percentile). This finding was consistent with thanatophoric dwarfism.

(Courtesy of the Perinatal Ultrasound Unit, Yale New Haven Medical Center, New Haven, Connecticut.)

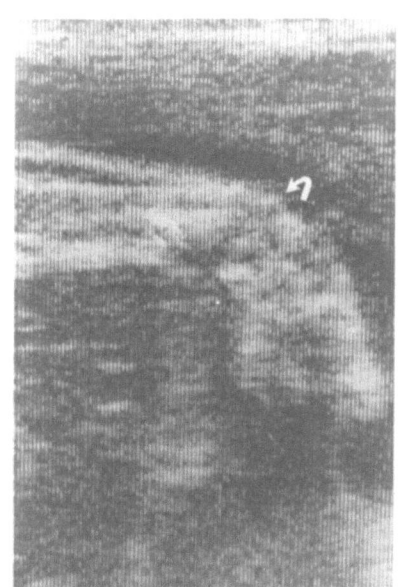

FIG. 17.7.2. CLUBFOOT

Longitudinal scan of the lower leg and foot demonstrating a clubfoot. Ankle (arrow). From Chervenak et al.[19]

Part II
Real-Time Sonography in Gynecology

Chapter 18
Principles of Gynecologic Sonography

- Gynecologic real-time sonography has entered routine office practice. Gynecologists who have had the opportunity to practice within a setting in which immediate sonographic evaluation is available will witness a major change in practice patterns.

- The limits of real-time sonography have, however, to be understood. Nothing is more dangerous than overinterpretation of sonographic findings. While the temptation may frequently exist, it must be recognized that sonography is not here to replace the pelvic examination but to serve as an adjunct to the pelvic examination.

- It is also important to note that sonography is not capable of making a histologic diagnosis. While certain sonographic findings may be suspicious, suggestive, or even indicative of a specific histopathologic lesion, sonography does not represent the appropriate tool to replace the microscope in histopathologic diagnosis.

- Thus, only if both its advantages and limitations are recognized will real-time sonography have the impact on gynecologic practice that it should have.

- For a sample report form, see Fig. 18.1.1.

GYNECOLOGIC
SONOGRAPHY REPORT

PATIENT'S NAME: _____

ADDRESS: _____

_____ Zip_____

TELEPHONE (Home): _____

TELEPHONE (Business): _____

DATE: _____

Referring Physician: _____

Address: _____

_____ Zip_____

Telephone: _____

Patient before: No _____ Yes _____

Patient Billing: _____ Office Billing: _____

AGE: _____ GRAVIDA: _____ PARA: _____ LMP: _____ EDC: _____

HX: _____ PREVIOUS SONO: Date: _____

Findings: _____

INDICATION FOR TEST: _____

SONOGRAPHIC RESULTS:

Uterus: Measures: _____ × _____ × _____cm

Homogeneous _____ Non-homogeneous _____

Location of Area: L_____ R_____

Measures:_____ × _____ × _____cm

Characteristics: Cystic_____Semi-solid_____Solid_____ Complex_____

Transonicity: Good_____ Fair_____Poor_____ None_____

Adnexa: Ovaries: Visualized L_____ Measures_____ × _____ × _____cm

R_____Measures_____ × _____ × _____cm

Homogeneous_____ Non-homogeneous_____

Mass: Located: L_____ R_____

Measures:_____ × _____ × _____cm

Characteristics: Cystic_____ Semi-solid_____ Solid_____Complex_____

Transonicity: Good_____Fair_____Poor_____None_____

COMMENTS: _____

_____

_____

_____

_____

_____

_____

Thank you for referring this patient. Should you have any further questions, please do not hesitate to call us.

M.D.

FIG. 18.1.1. SAMPLE GYNECOLOGIC SONOGRAPHY REPORT FORM

Chapter 19
Normal Pelvic Anatomy

19.1. PRINCIPLES

- Gynecologic scans always require a full bladder as an acoustic window.

- Consequently, pelvic structures will be sonographically visible by oblique scanning by either of two methods:

  o Transducer follows an oblique axis (see Fig. 19.1.1).
  o The patient is rotated obliquely.

- In contrast to static scanning, exact slicing of the body cannot be achieved with real-time sonography. It is therefore crucial to define all normal pelvic structures as a first step in every gynecologic scan.

- It is either the recognition of the absence of a normal structure or the addition of yet another structure to the normal expected entities of the pelvis that allows for the diagnosis of an abnormality.

- Although standards have not yet been established, we and clinicians at many other centers describe sonographic locations by the following parameters:
  LO = midline   L(+) = right side   L(−) = left side
          P(+) = above symphysis pubis

  Example:

  L(+)4, P(+)7–8 represents an entity 4 cm to right of the midline, 7–8 cm above symphysis pubis (see Fig. 19.1.2).

19.2. PELVIC ORGANS

The recommended sequence in performing a pelvic scan begins with a *longitudinal midline scan,* followed by *longitudinal oblique adnexal scanning* on each side (see Fig. 19.1.1) and *transverse scans* starting at the symphysis pubis and moving cephalad.

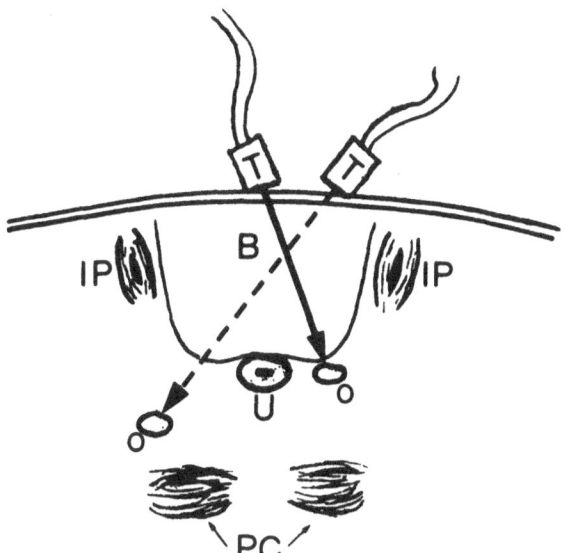

FIG. 19.1.1. PRINCIPLE OF THE ACOUSTIC WINDOW

Schematic illustration of the acoustic window technique performed by angling from the midline (solid arrow) or by using the entire bladder from the opposite side (broken arrow). The patient can also be angled such that the bladder can be utilized with a normal transducer angle. Bladder (B), iliopsoas (IP), ovary (o), pubococcygeal (PC), uterus (U), transducer (T). (Illustration by R. V. Giglia.)

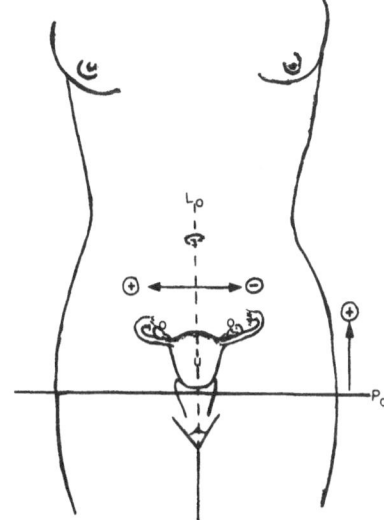

FIG. 19.1.2. SCHEME FOR GEOGRAPHIC COORDINATES IN GYNECOLOGIC SCANNING

Longitudinal (L), symphysis pubis (P_o), uterus (u), ovary (o).

19.2.1. Longitudinal Midline Scan

- Performing a longitudinal midline scan permits identification of an adequately filled bladder, which should always cover the uterine fundus.

- This scan should be performed in the abdominal midline with the umbilicus as a reference point, thereby permitting recognition of deviated and absent uteri (see Fig. 19.2.1).

- The angle of the transducer should be perpendicular to the structure to be identified, e.g., the transducer angle will vary with position of the uterus (see Fig. 19.2.2).

- *The uterus*
  - Normal dimensions are approximately 8 × 4 × 3.5 cm.
  - Variations of uterine size, however, should be taken into account depending on age, parity, and shape in pre- or postmenopausal stages (see Fig. 19.2.3).
  - The sonographic appearance:
    Homogeneous (similar to liver parenchyma)
    Well defined, smooth, with a continuous outline
    Central linear echo (endometrial cavity)
    Anteverted uterus: along posterior bladder wall (see Fig. 19.2.2A)
    Retroverted uterus: away from bladder (see Fig. 19.2.2B)

- *The cervix* is difficult to visualize sonographically.

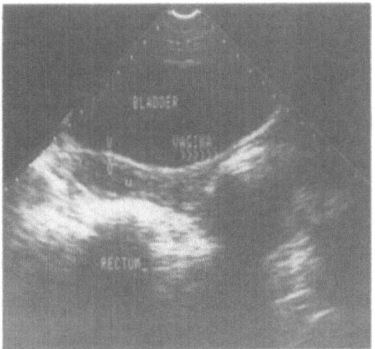

FIG. 19.2.1. NORMAL LONGITUDINAL MIDLINE SCAN

Longitudinal sector scan of normal midline structures. Uterus (u), endometrial echo (arrowheads).

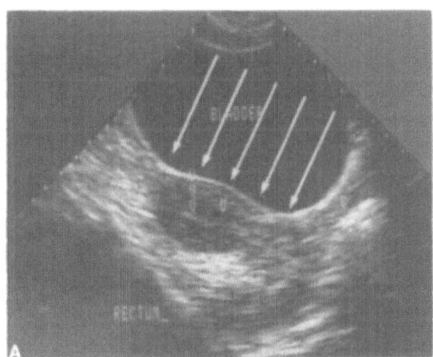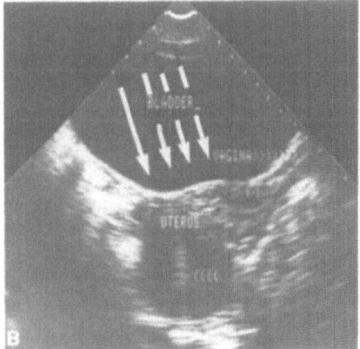

FIG. 19.2.2. ANGLE OF INCIDENCE (TRANSDUCER) IN PELVIC SCAN OF ANTEVERTED AND RETROVERTED UTERI

Sector scan of the angle of the ultrasound beam (arrows) to visualize an anteverted (A) and retroverted (B) uterus. Endometrial echo (arrowheads).

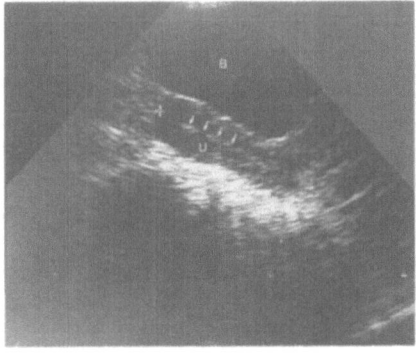

FIG. 19.2.3. NORMAL SONOGRAPHIC APPEARANCE OF UTERUS

Normal uterus in the longitudinal midline scan. Note the homogeneity, smooth borders, and slight increase in the endometrial echo (arrows). Uterus (U), bladder (B).

CHAPTER 19 • NORMAL PELVIC ANATOMY

- *The vagina*
  - ○ The sonographic appearance:
    - Linear, double-contour structure with increased central echoes
    - Defined anteriorly by the bladder
  - ○ *Anteverted uterus*: the uterine position follows the posterior contour of the bladder. (The angle between vagina and central uterine axis is approximately 135°.) (see Fig. 19.2.4A).
  - ○ *Retroverted uterus*: this angle is larger than 180°, whereas the angle with the posterior contour of the bladder remains at approximately 135°. (see Fig. 19.2.4B).

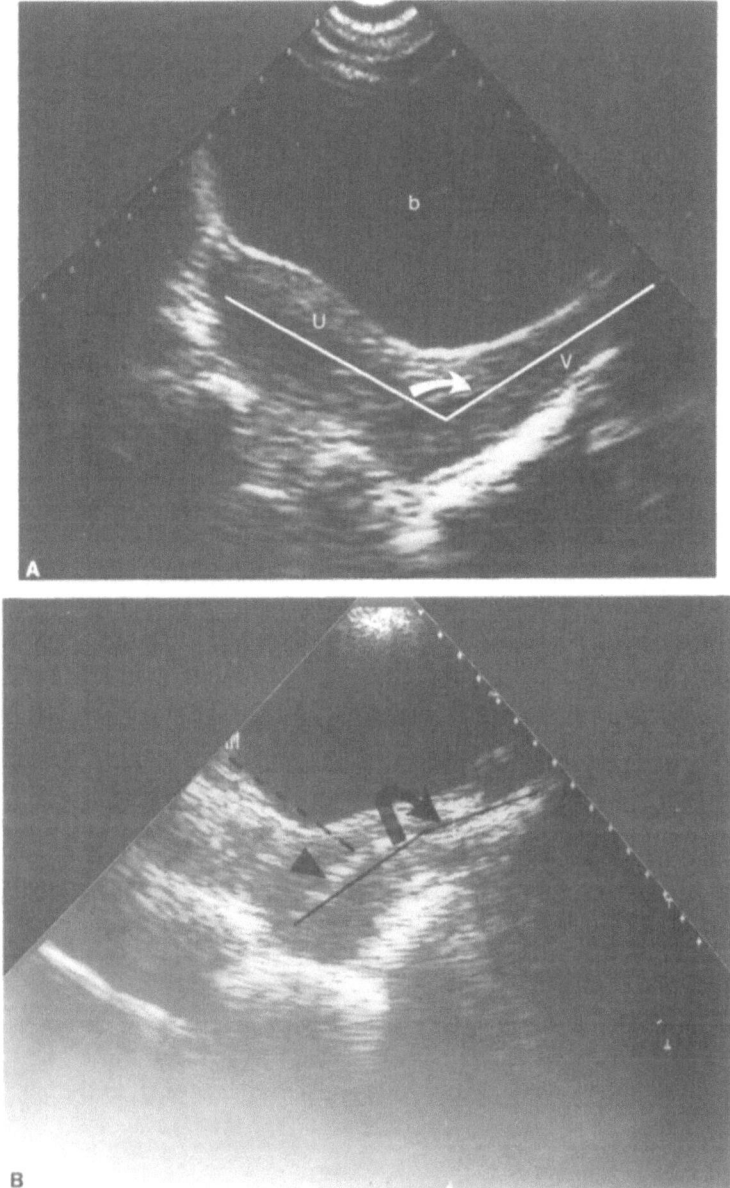

FIG. 19.2.4. THE RELATIONSHIP AMONG VAGINA, BLADDER, AND ANTEVERTED AS WELL AS RETROVERTED

UTERI

(A)   The angle (arrow) of the vagina (V) to the anteverted uterus (U) is approximately 135°. Bladder (b).

(B)   The angle (arrow) of the vagina (V) to the retroverted uterus (U) is greater than 180°. The bladder (b) remains at approximately 135° (dotted line); intrauterine device (arrowhead).

- *The cul-de-sac* represents the lowest point within the pelvic cavity.

    o Sonographically it is represented by the area posterior to the uterovaginal junction (cervix) and anterior to the rectum (see Fig. 19.2.5).
    o This is the area in which peritoneal fluid accumulates; it is visible sonographically.
    o Only if fluid is present will the cul-de-sac be visible sonographically.

- *The rectum* lies posterior to the above structures (see Fig. 19.2.6).

    o Real-time sonography has made identification of the intestinal tract relatively simple due to recognition of *peristaltic activity.*
    o This may preclude the still widely employed practice of rectal and intestinal identification with water contrast (enema) of the rectum.[1]

REFERENCE

1. Kurtz AB, Rifkin MD: Normal anatomy of the female pelvis, in Callen PW (ed): *Ultrasonography in Obstetrics and Gynecology.* Philadelphia, WB Saunders, 1983, pp 193–208.

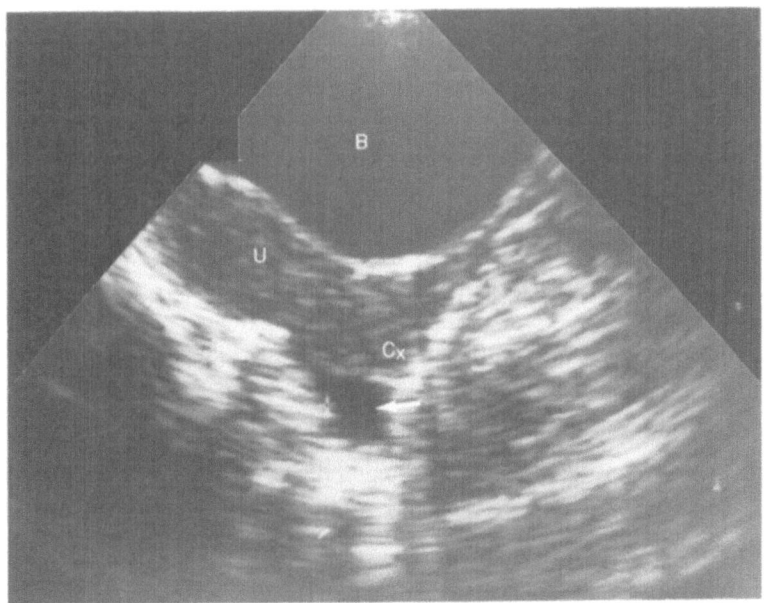

FIG. 19.2.5. CUL-DE-SAC FLUID

Fluid in the cul-de-sac (arrow). Note its irregular shape and the absence of clear borders. Bladder (B), uterus (U), cervix (Cx).

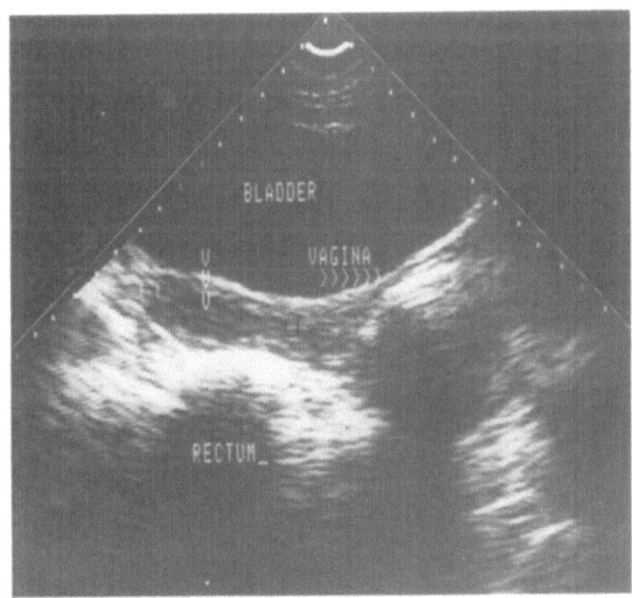

FIG. 19.2.6. THE RECTUM

Longitudinal scan depicting the typical appearance of the rectum posterior to the uterus (u). Note the blockage of the ultrasound beam due to the air in the rectum.

19.2.2. Longitudinal Oblique Scan

- These scans can be obtained by oblique rotation of either the transducer or the patient. This is done in order to use the acoustic window of the bladder (see Section 19.1 and Fig. 19.1.2).

- In most cases, oblique rotation of the transducer will represent the easier alternative. However, when it becomes necessary to investigate the presence of fluid levels, oblique rotation of the patient becomes essential.

- *The ovary*
  The normal ovary is located laterally to the uterus and is free floating (see Fig. 19.2.7).

  o The normal size of an ovary is approximately $3 \times 2 \times 1$ cm. However, ovarian size will vary with time of the menstrual cycle, age and pre- and postmenopausal stages.[2]
  o The nonfollicular ovary has a sonographic appearance similar to that of the uterus. It is homogeneous and has a smooth, *almond-shaped* contour.
  o The formation of follicular cysts represents a normal cyclic process (see Fig. 19.2.8). A detailed discussion is presented in Chapter 20, Follicular Sonography.
  o The ovary will not always be sonographically apparent. Lack of its identification will, however, support the contention that no abnormal enlargement is present. Clinical correlation is crucial in such cases.

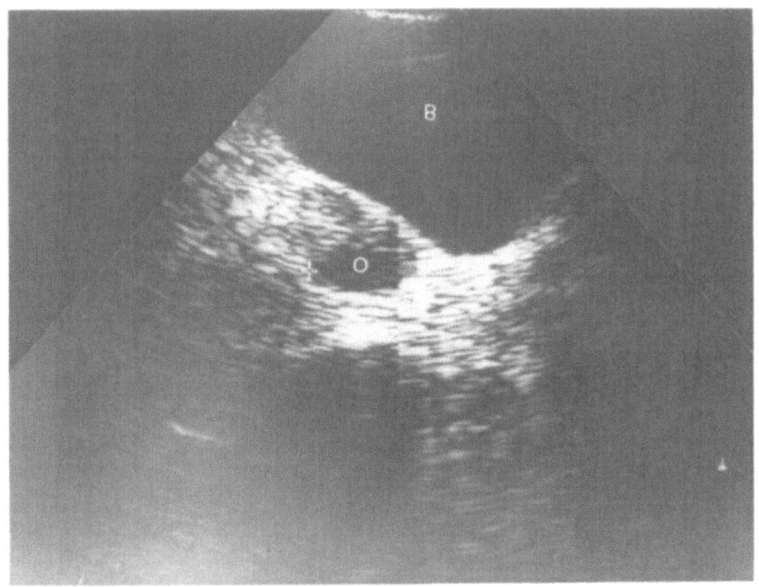

FIG. 19.2.7. NORMAL OVARY

Longitudinal oblique scan of a normal ovary (O). Note its homogeneity and almond shape. Bladder (B).

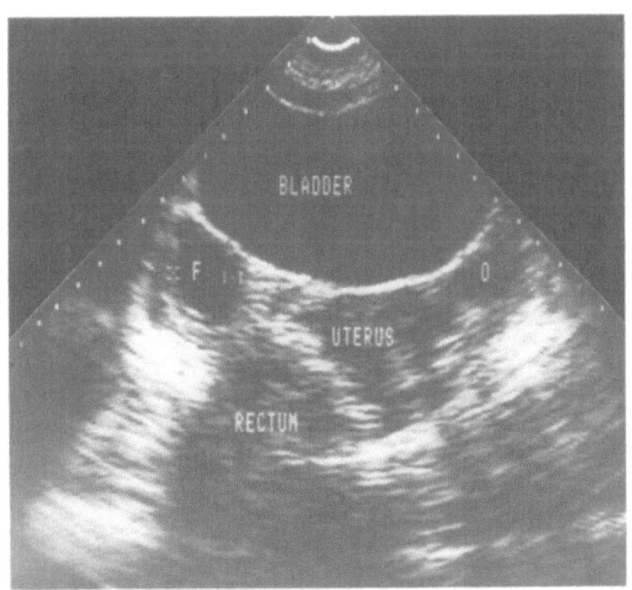

FIG. 19.2.8. SPONTANEOUS OVULATORY CYCLE

Transverse sector scan demonstrating a normal follicle (F). The opposite ovary (O) is visualized and appears within normal limits.

19.2.3. Transverse Scan

- *Pelvic musculature*

    Identification of individual pelvic muscles is particularly important in their differential diagnosis from pelvic masses.

    o The following muscles are identified most commonly (see Figs. 19.2.9 and 19.2.10):

    Iliopsoas muscles
    Obturator internus muscles
    Pubococcygeal muscles

    o Most of these muscles are more easily identifiable in a transverse scan. Their identification may vary from individual to individual.

    o The differential diagnosis of pelvic muscles from masses is aided by the fact that muscle groups usually are identifiable in a very symmetric pattern, bilaterally.

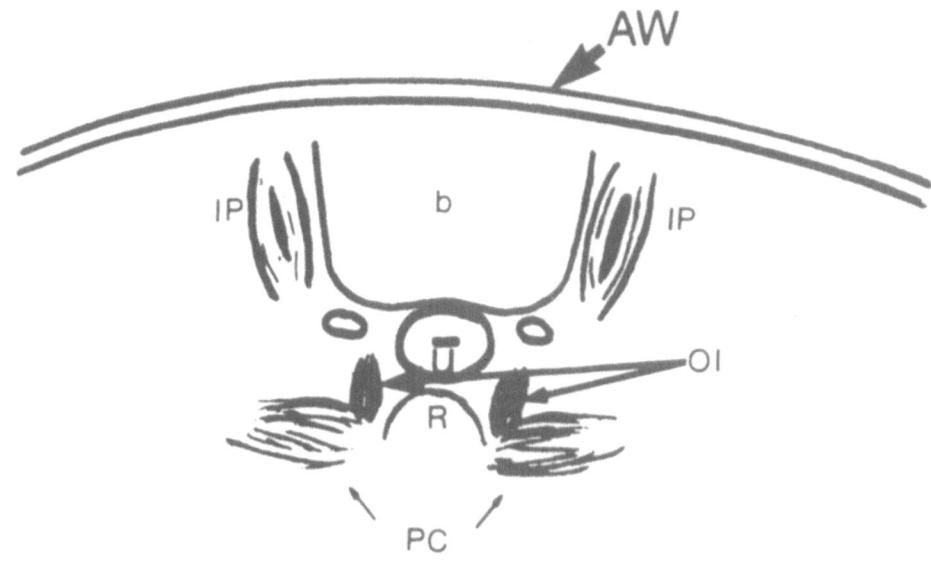

FIG. 19.2.9. PELVIC MUSCLE GROUPS

Schemation illustration of the normal location of the pelvic musculature visualized on a transverse scan. Abdominal wall (AW), bladder (b), iliopsoas (IP), uterus (U), obturator internis (OI), rectum (R), and pubococcygeal (PC). (Illustration by R. V. Giglia.)

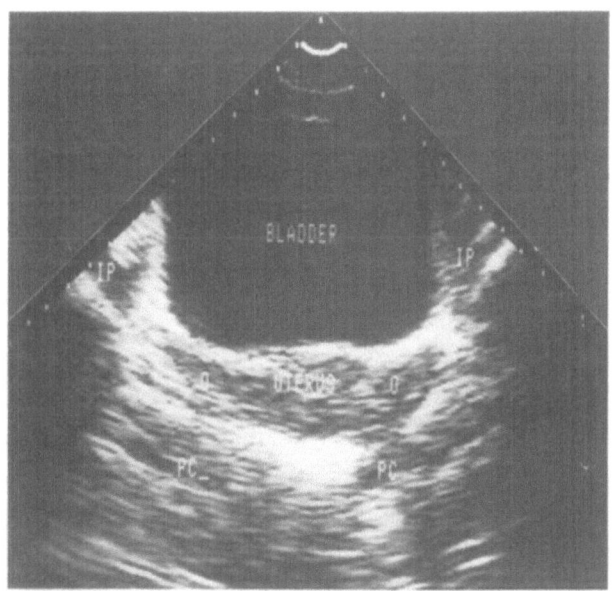

FIG. 19.2.10. PELVIC MUSCULATURE

Transverse sector scan of the pelvic muscles. Iliopsoas (IP), ovary (O), pubococcygeal (PC).

- *Uterus*

     The uterus is typically located centrally below the bladder.

     o The sonographic appearance should be homogeneous with a central linear echo, representing the endometrial cavity. The uterus should have a smooth and clear outline (see Fig. 19.2.11).

- *The adnexae*
     Normal tubes and round ligaments can only rarely be clearly visualized.

- *The ovaries*
     Normal ovaries are usually located lateral to the uterine corpus immediately below the filled bladder. Alterations from this position of the ovaries may be normal but should be cause for suspicion of pelvic pathology, primarily adhesion formation (see Fig. 19.2.11).

- *The bladder*
     Centrally located, the bladder has a smooth symetrically thin contour (see Fig. 19.2.12). Abnormal thickening of the bladder or internal echoes should be cause for suspicion of bladder pathology.

REFERENCES

2. Campbell S, Goessens L, Goswamy R, et al: Realtime ultrasonography for determination of ovarian morphology and volume. *Lancet* 1982;1:145.

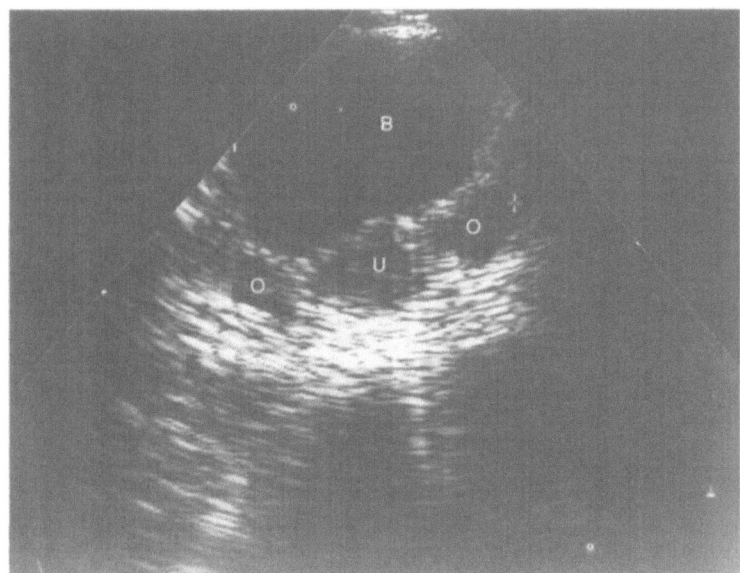

FIG. 19.2.11. UTERUS AND OVARIES

Transverse sector scan of the normal position of the uterus (U) and ovaries (O). Bladder (B).

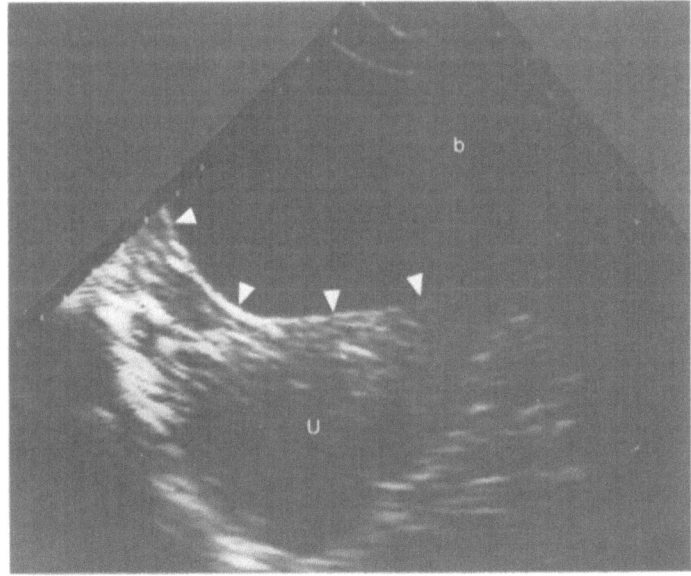

FIG. 19.2.12. BLADDER WALL

Longitudinal sector scan visualizing the normal appearance of the posterior wall (arrowheads). Note the smooth contour. Any variation in thickness or the smooth appearance should be considered abnormal. Uterus (U), bladder (b).

Chapter 20
Follicular Sonography

- Follicular sonography (FS) has revolutionized the fertility practice[1-3] and probably represents one of the most decisive factors in the rapid and successful evolution of in vitro fertilization.

- Follicular sonography may be applied either during natural cycles (in most instances only one dominant follicle occurs) or during stimulated cycles, in which multiple follicles need to be followed. In both cases, a baseline scan may be performed to rule out major pathology.

20.1. THE NATURAL CYCLE

20.1.1. Indications for Sonography

Sonography during a natural cycle may be used for any of the following indications:

- Confirmation of ovulation

- Evaluation of natural follicular size

- Unruptured follicle syndrome

- Ovulation timing for artificial insemination, human chorionic gonadotropin (hCG) therapy, etc.

20.1.2. The Normal Follicle

- Follicles are located peripherally within the ovary

- Their appearance is cystic with thin, well-defined smooth borders and good transonicity (see Figs. 20.1.1–20.1.3).

- Follicular measurements should be made of all three diameters of the follicle. Some centers report follicles according to largest diameter, while others establish the mean of all three parameters.

- Normal growth for the dominant follicle is usually rapid and may grow as much as 5 mm/day during the preovulatory phase.

- Nondominant follicles usually grow significantly slower and may arrest or even degenerate before ovulation.

- The normal preovulatory follicle in a natural cycle usually reach 20–25 mm but may have a wider range of 15–30 mm.

- Particularly when follicles reach a diameter of more than 25 mm the differentiation from a functional cyst may be difficult.

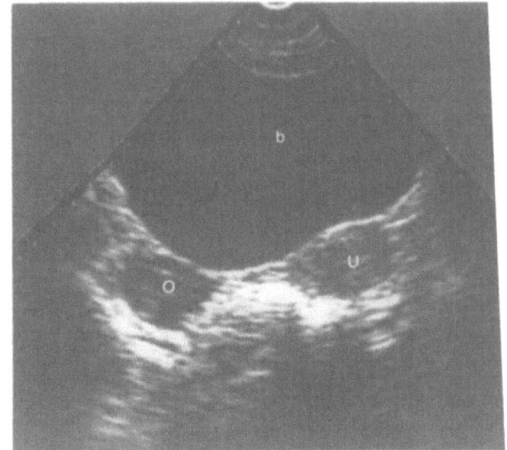

FIG. 20.1.1. FOLLICULAR DEVELOPMENT

Transverse sector scan demonstrating the beginning of follicular development in the natural cycle. Note the enlarged ovary (O) with some changes in the normal homogeneous appearance. Bladder (b), uterus (u).

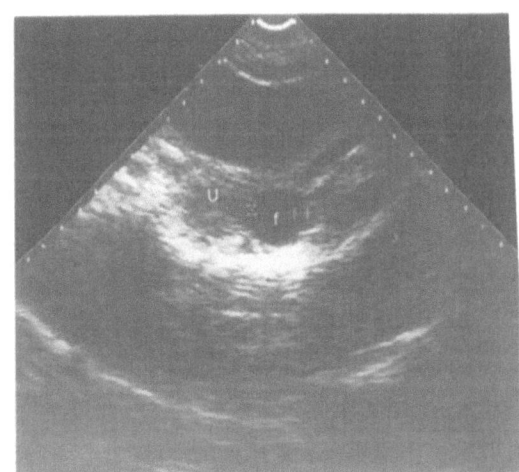

FIG. 20.1.2. TYPICAL FOLLICLE

Transverse sector scan of the typical appearance of a follicle (f) in a natural cycle. Uterus (U).

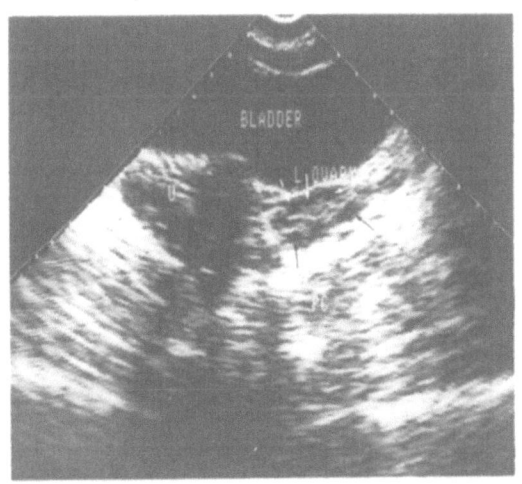

FIG. 20.1.3. MULTIPLE FOLLICULAR FORMATIONS

Transverse scan of the left ovary. Note the areas of decreased echogenicity within the ovary. Multiple follicle formation (arrows). Uterus (U), pubococcygeal muscle (PC).

CHAPTER 20 • FOLLICULAR SONOGRAPHY **187**

20.1.3. Ovulation

- Sonographic evidence of ovulation consists of the following findings:
    - Reduction in size or disappearance of a dominant follicle
    - Disappearance of clear cystic space or appearance of internal echoes, or both
    - Loss of smoothness of follicular borders with separation of lining (*crenation*)[4] (see Fig. 20.1.4A)
    - Excessive fluid in cul de sac
    - Leaking follicles demonstrating fluid tracks (Fig. 20.1.4B)

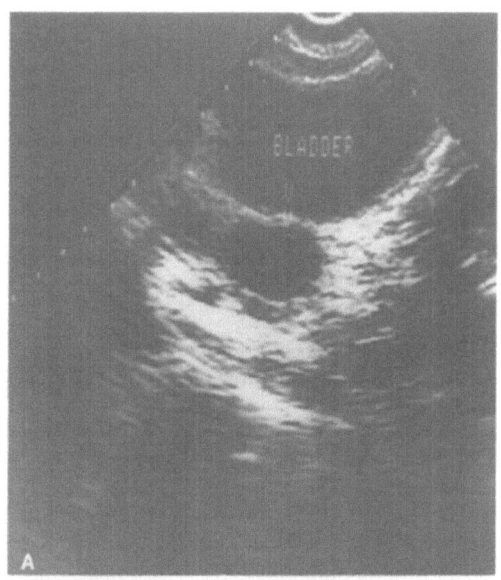

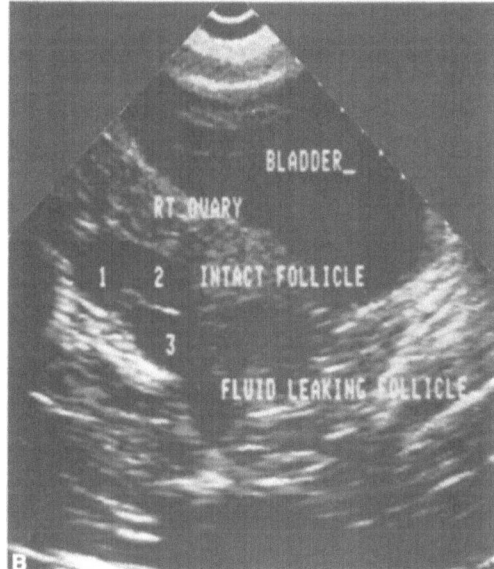

FIG. 20.1.4. SONOGRAPHIC EVIDENCE OF OVULATION

(A)   Sonographic picture of imminent ovulation. Arrows point to the areas of crenation seen within the follicular wall.

(B)   Leaking fluid from a follicle is a sign of ovulation.

20.2. THE INDUCED CYCLE

- Ovulatory cycles may be induced with either clomiphene citrate (Clomid) or human menopausal gonadotropin (hMG) (Pergonal).

- Both medications will induce multiple follicles; however, a larger number will be induced with hMG than with Clomid (see Fig. 20.2.1).

- A difference will also be apparent in preovulatory follicular size between these two medications. In a Clomid-stimulated cycle one, but preferably two, follicles of 18–25 mm diameter should be seen before hCG-induced ovulation, while in a Pergonal-stimulated cycle preferably two follicles of 16–17 mm are to be seen before hCG administration.

20.2.1. Indications for Sonography

Sonography during a stimulated cycle may be indicated for the following:

- Ovulation induction with Clomid
- Ovulation induction with Pergonal
- Artificial insemination in stimulated cycle
- In vitro fertilization (IVF)

20.2.2. The Stimulated Follicle

With the exception of number of follicles and preovulatory size differences, no important sonographic distinctions can be seen between stimulated and natural follicles. Technically, however, multiple follicles are more difficult to discern.

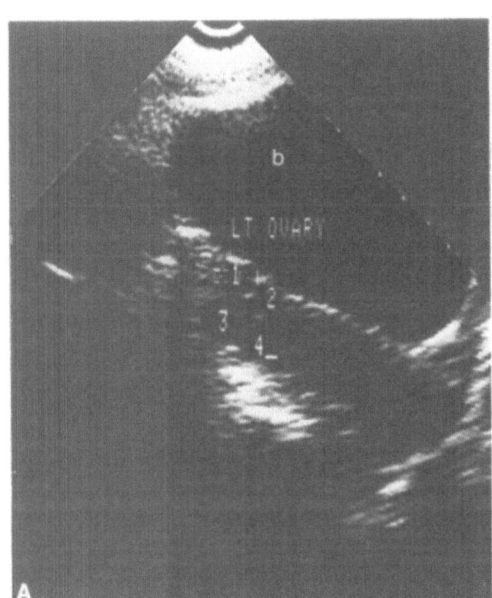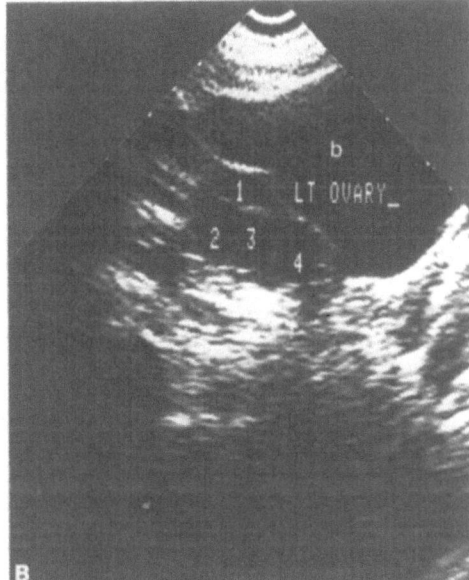

FIG. 20.2.1. FOLLICULAR GROWTH PATTERN DURING A STIMULATED CYCLE

(A) Early follicular development shown in a longitudinal scan of the left ovary (four follicles).

(B) Serial scan of follicular development showing the increase in size as well as the clearer definition. Bladder (b).

20.2.3. Ovulation

- The sonographic picture of ovulation in a stimulated cycle is not different from the signs described for the natural cycle (see Fig. 20.1.4).

- Reporting of stimulated cycle sonography may be documented on a single report sheet to permit a quick and simple review of the stimulation process. A sample sheet is presented in Fig. 20.2.2.

FOLLICULAR SONOGRAPHY REPORT

TO BE FILLED OUT BY REFERRING PHYSICIAN

PATIENT'S NAME: ____________________

ADDRESS: ____________________

____________________ Zip ____________________

TELEPHONE (Home): ____________________

TELEPHONE (Business): ____________________

DATE: ____________________

Referring Physician: ____________________

Address: ____________________

____________________ Zip ____________________

Telephone: ____________________

Patient before: No ______ Yes ______

Patient Billing: ______ Office Billing: ______

AGE: ____________ PARA: ____________ LMP: ____________

HX: ____________________

TO BE RECORDED BY PERINATAL TESTING CENTER

FOLLICLE GROWTH — R Ovary — L Ovary

1. Date: ____________________
   Number of Follicles: ____________ Number of Follicles: ____________
   Comments: ____________ Comments: ____________

2. Date: ____________________
   Number of Follicles: ____________ Number of Follicles: ____________
   Comments: ____________ Comments: ____________

3. Date: ____________________
   Number of Follicles: ____________ Number of Follicles: ____________
   Comments: ____________ Comments: ____________

4. Date: ____________________
   Number of Follicles: ____________ Number of Follicles: ____________
   Comments: ____________ Comments: ____________

5. Date: ____________________
   Number of Follicles: ____________ Number of Follicles: ____________
   Comments: ____________ Comments: ____________

COMMENTS: ____________________

Thank you for referring this patient. Should you have any further questions, please do not hesitate to call us.

____________________ M.D.

FIG. 20.2.2. SAMPLE FOLLICULAR SONOGRAPHY REPORT

20.3. SONOGRAPHIC EGG RETRIEVAL FOR IVF

Sonographic egg retrieval was reported in 1983 using primarily two alternative approaches:

20.3.1. Transabdominal (Transvesicle) Approach[5,6]

- Under sonographic guidance, a long aspiration needle is inserted at a 60° angle through the abdominal wall and the filled bladder toward the underlying ovary into the follicle(s) (see Fig. 20.3.1).

- This approach is best suited for the patient with normally located ovaries (i.e., immediately beneath the bladder).

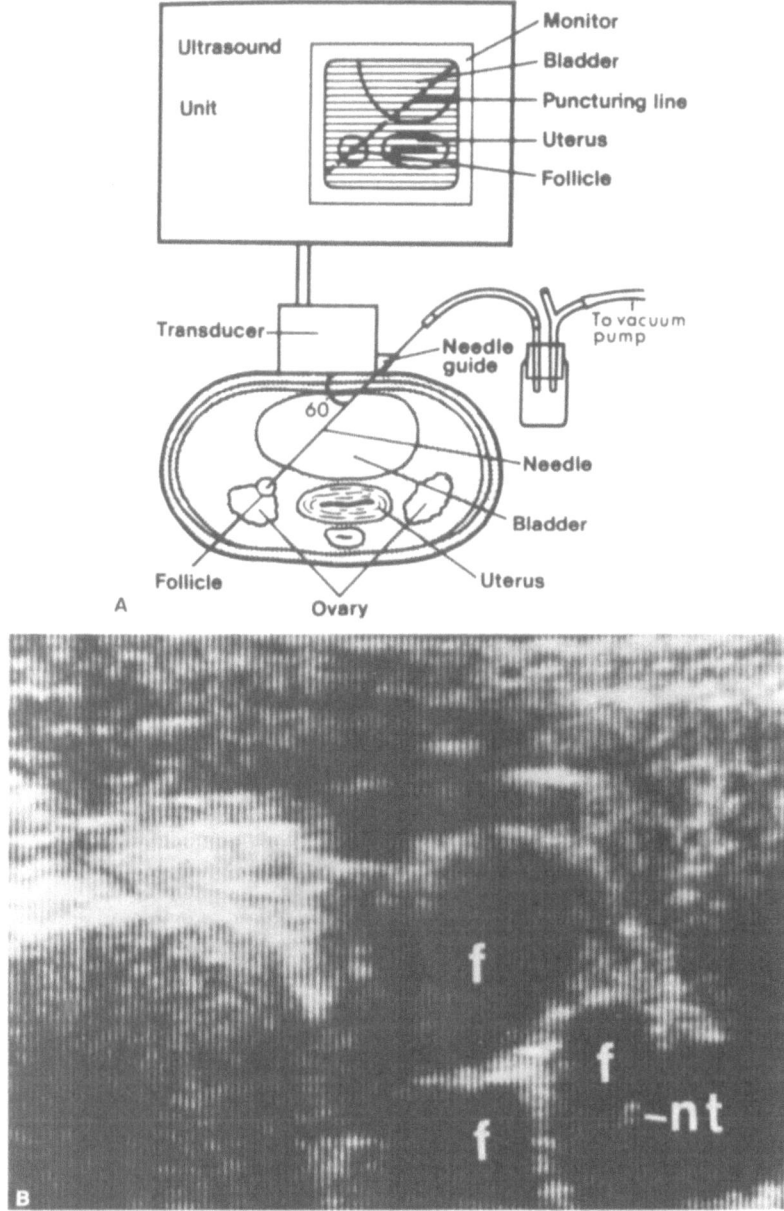

FIG. 20.3.1. TRANSABDOMINAL SONOGRAPHIC EGG RETRIEVAL FOR IVF

(A) Schematic illustration of the ultrasonically guided puncture technique.

(B) Illustration of ultrasonically guided puncture of a human follicle. The white echo inside the follicle (f) represents the needle tip (nt).
From Wikland et al.[6]

20.3.2. Transvaginal Approach[7]

- Under sonographic guidance, a long aspiration needle is inserted via the posterior fornix of the vagina into the cul-de-sac and directed toward the ovary and follicle(s) (see Fig. 20.3.2).

- This approach is best suited for the patient in whom adhesions have fixed an ovary into the cul-de-sac.

- Sonographic egg retrieval for IVF has been found to be a safe and cost-effective method that allows IVF to be performed as an ambulatory office procedure.

REFERENCES

1. Hackelöer B, Fleming R, Robinson H, et al: Correlation of ultrasonic and endocrinologic assessment of human follicular development. *Am J Obstet Gynecol* 1979;135:122.
2. O'Herliky L, deCrespigney L, Copato A, et al: Preovulatory follicular size: A comparison of ultrasound and laparoscopic measurements. *Fertil Steril* 1980;34:24.
3. Smith D, Picker R, Simosich P: Assessment of ovulation by ultrasound and estradiol levels during spontaneous and induced cycles. *Fertil Steril* 1980;33:387.
4. Picker R, Smith D, Tucker M, et al: Ultrasonic signs of imminent ovulation. *J Clin Ultrasound* 1983;11:1.
5. Lenz S, Lauritsen JG: Ultrasonically guided percutaneous aspiration of human follicles under local anesthesia: A new method of collecting oocytes for in vitro fertilization. *Fertil Steril* 1982;38:673.
6. Wikland M, Nilsson L, Hansson R, et al: Collection of human oocytes by the use of sonography. *Fertil Steril* 1983;39:603.
7. Gleicher, N, Friberg J, Fullan N, et al: Egg retrieval for in vitro fertilization by sonographically controlled vaginal culdocentesis. *Lancet* 1983;2:508.

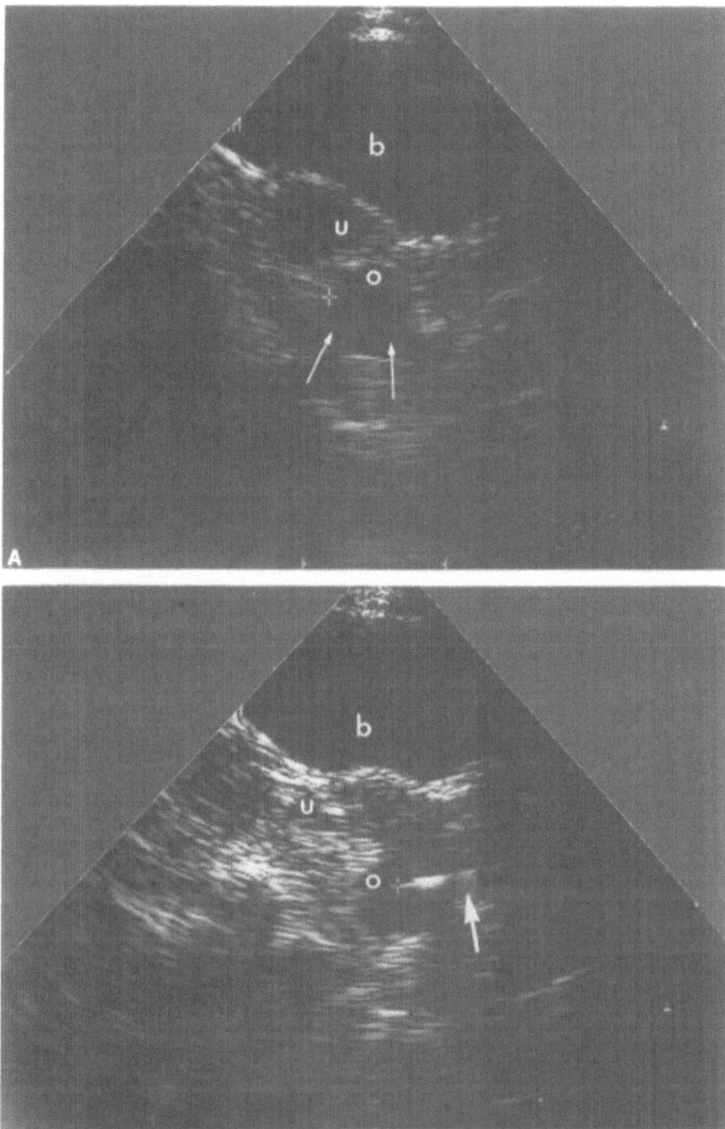

FIG. 20.3.2. TRANSVAGINAL SONOGRAPHIC EGG RETRIEVAL FOR IVF

(A) Longitudinal scan (L-2) to localize the ovary and follicle for transvaginal egg retrieval. Bladder (b), uterus (u), ovary (o), follicles (arrows).

(B) Longitudinal scan (L-2) showing the penetration of the follicle by the aspiration needle (arrow). Bladder (b), uterus (u), ovary (o).

Chapter 21
Abnormal Pelvic Anatomy

21.1. UTERINE ABNORMALITIES

21.1.1. Congenital Abnormalities

- Congenital abnormalities of the uterus may represent a wide spectrum from congenital absence of the uterus, rudimentary uterus, didelphys, and bicornis (see Figs. 21.1.1 and 21.1.2) to lesser abnormalities such as uterus subseptus, septus, or arcuatus.

- Most of these congenital abnormalities of the uterus have been diagnosed sonographically.

- Other reported abnormalities include blind uterine horn with or without connection to the remaining uterine corpus, T-shaped and *hypoplastic* when in conjunction with diethylstilbestrol (DES) exposure, as well as other minor disorders.

- Ultrasound has also been helpful in the performance of first trimester abortions in patients with double cervix and double uteri. Entry into the gestational cavity may at times only be possible with sonographic guidance (Giglia and Gleicher, personal communication).

21.1.2. Uterine Myomas

- Except for pregnancy, uterine myomas represent the most frequent cause for uterine enlargement.

- Uterine myomas can be detected by ultrasound in almost all instances.

- Ultrasound permits accurate assessment of size, localization, and assessment of internal characteristics such as calcification and cystic degeneration (see Fig. 21.1.3).

- Ultrasound also frequently permits the differential diagnosis between a uterine myoma and an adnexal mass—but such differentiation must be performed with caution.

- A pedunculated myoma is at times difficult to differentiate from an adnexal mass.

- Sarcomas cannot be differentiated sonographically from benign myomas.

- The ultrasonic appearance of a myoma will be nonhomogeneous in most instances. Fibroids with calcifications may produce acoustic shadowing. The uterus cannot be separated from the myoma; transonicity will be decreased and uterine borders may become irregular. Myomas may distort the posterior bladder wall.

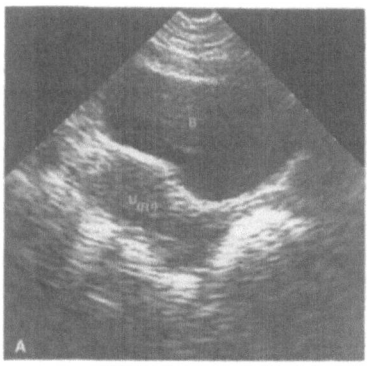 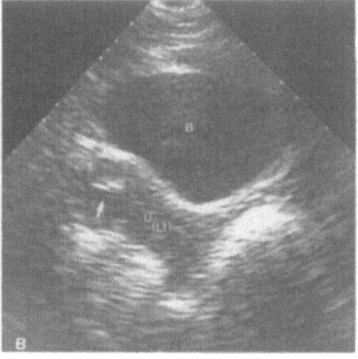

FIG. 21.1.1. BICORNUATE UTERUS

Longitudinal scans of right and left horns of a bicornuate uterus. Arrow in left horn points to calcified area. Bladder (B), uterus (U), left (LT), right (RT).

FIG. 21.1.2. BICORNUATE UTERUS

Transverse scan in the fundal portion of bicornuate uterus. Arrow points to calcified area in left horn.

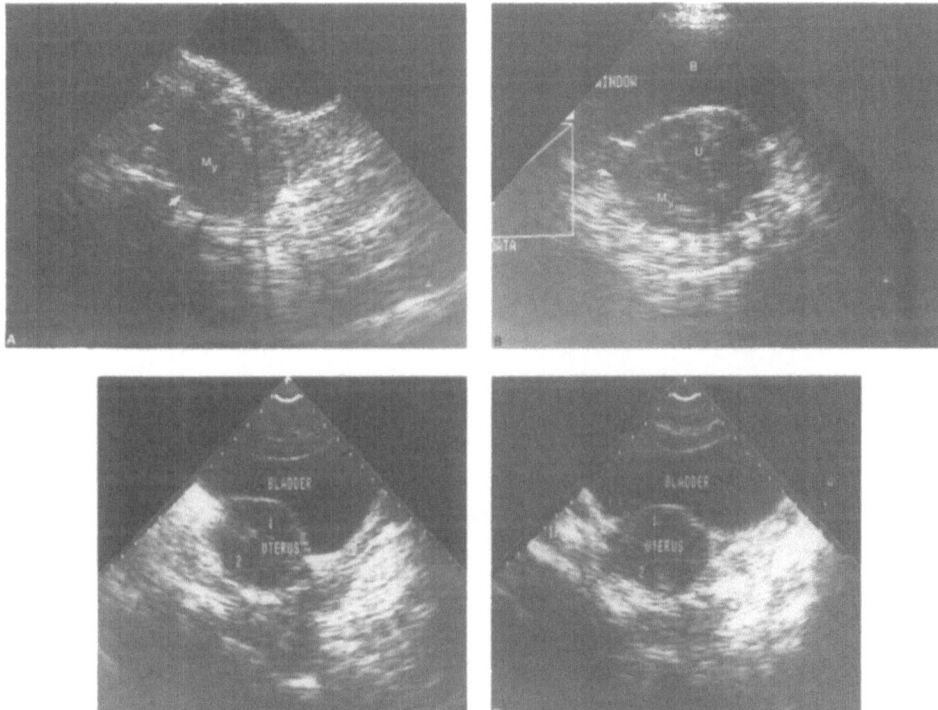

FIG. 21.1.3. UTERINE MYOMAS

Longitudinal (A) and transverse (B) scans of a posterior fibroid (My). Note the nonhomogeneity and bulging of the border (arrows). Normal uterine (U) tissue is seen anterior to the myoma (MY). Bladder (B).

Longitudinal (C) and transverse (D) scans of multiple fibroid uterus. The areas of nonhomogeneity are indicated by 1 and 2. Vagina (V), iliopsoas (IP).

21.1.3. Intrauterine Devices

- Sonography has become particularly helpful in evaluating the so-called lost IUD.

- Sonography may be used to locate the IUD and may be used in its retrieval by directing a retrieval instrument under sonographic guidance into the endometrial cavity.

- The vast majority of IUDs will be sonographically visible if within the uterine cavity, particularly those that contain copper.

- Lost IUDs within the peritoneal cavity cannot reliably be located by means of sonography and should be evaluated with standard x-ray film of the pelvis.

- The ultrasonic appearance of IUDs will vary with the product:

  o Lippes Loops give a dotted appearance in the longitudinal axis due to their tortuosity (see Fig. 21.1.4).
  o The Cu-7 will appear longitudinally as a bright continuous midline echo (see Fig. 21.1.4).

Both IUDs will be sonographically bright reflectors and, contrary to endometrial echoes, will not disappear at low gain.

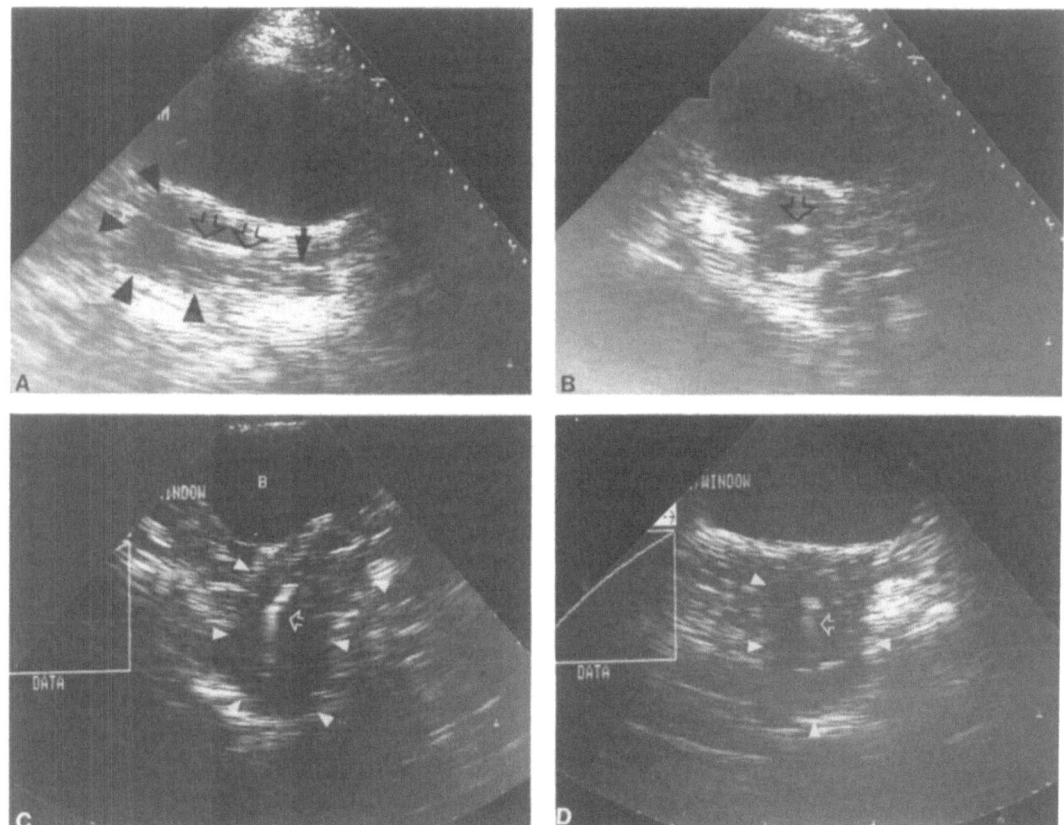

FIG. 21.1.4.   INTRAUTERINE DEVICES (IUD)

Longitudinal (A) and transverse (B) sector scan of a centrally located IUD (open arrow) in an anteverted uterus (arrowheads). Note the abnormally low position of the IUD in the cervical region (arrow).

Longitudinal (C) and transverse (D) sector scan of a centrally located IUD (open arrowheads) in a retroverted uterus (solid arrowheads). Note the characteristic increase in echoes from the IUD. Bladder (B).

21.2. ADNEXAL PATHOLOGY

21.2.1. Tubal Abnormalities

- Sonographically detectable tubal pathology will be largely reflective of two disease states: *pelvic inflammatory disease (PID)* and *endometriosis.*

- The use of real-time sonography for these two disease states is limited. The sonographic diagnosis is restricted to a description of anatomic consequences of these diseases on the pelvic anatomy. Tubal pathology, in particular, may look sonographically identical in both PID and endometriosis.

- The sonographic appearance of these two diseases will depend on the severity of the individual entity. Excluding more specific findings, such as *tubo-ovarian abscesses (TOA)* and *endometriomas* (Sections 21.2.2 and 21.2.4), sonographic findings will be nonspecific and include the following:

  o Disorganized sonographic picture of the adnexae, which prohibits differentiation and recognition of normal pelvic structures (see Chapter 19 and Fig. 21.2.1).

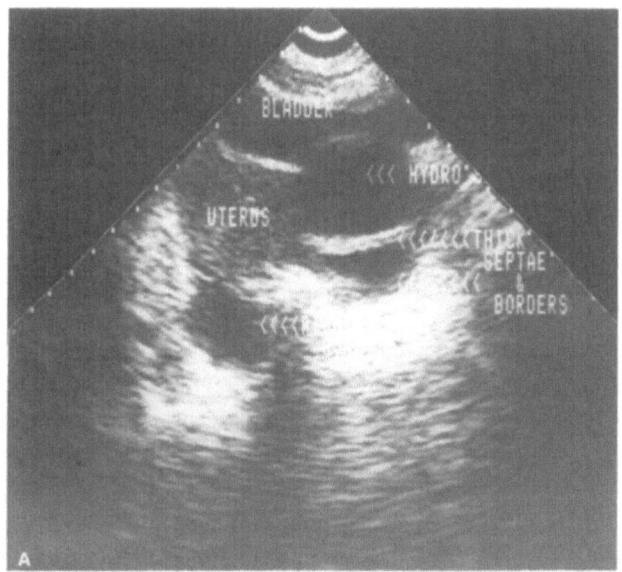

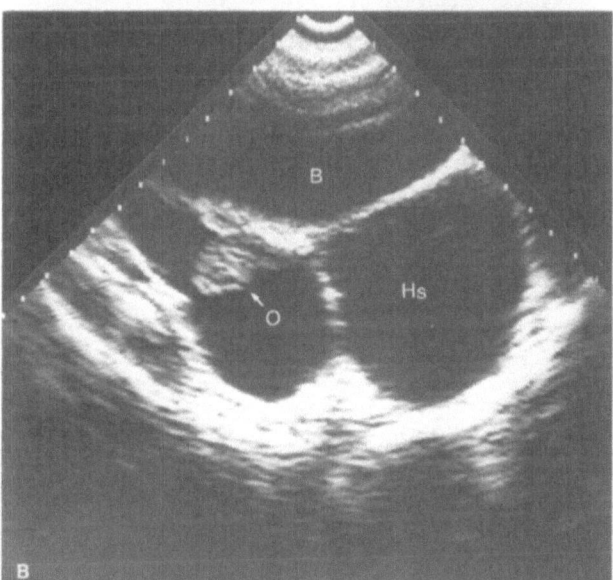

FIG. 21.2.1. PELVIC INFLAMMATORY DISEASE (PID)

(A) Transverse sector scan depicting the sonographic appearance of acute PID. Note the thick borders and septae as well as the difficulty in visualizing exact borders. Hydrosalpinx (HYDRO).

(B) Transverse sector scan illustrating acute inflammation of the tubes (Hs). Note the mainly cystic appearance, which can be misdiagnosed as a multiloculated ovarian cyst. Bladder (B), ovary (O).

o *In the more acute phase* of an inflammatory pelvic process, cystic spaces, lined by thick borders and interrupted with thick septae, are characteristic and can give the sonographic appearance of a multiloculated cyst (see Fig. 21.2.2).

o Characteristically, the cul de sac is involved in this process in both diseases.

o *In the more chronic phase* of PID, differentiation from endometriosis becomes even more difficult. Because of organization and degeneration, the sonographic picture becomes even more complex, resulting in a diffuse and more bizarre appearance. This appearance is characterized by sonolucent and sonodense areas that may cause acoustic shadowing. The ovaries are difficult to identify; as a result, the differential diagnosis from an adnexal mass may be tricky (see Fig. 21.2.3).

o An organized *tubo-ovarian abscess (TOA)* may be sonographically similar to the above-described chronic process. It will frequently, however, have clearer defined borders, and *fluid levels* may be seen within individual cystic spaces. These fluid levels can be identified by means of the technique of tilting the patient (see Chapter 19.1). In whichever direction the patient is tilted with real-time sonography, the flow of the intracavitary fluid into the horizontal plane can be visualized (see Fig. 21.2.4).

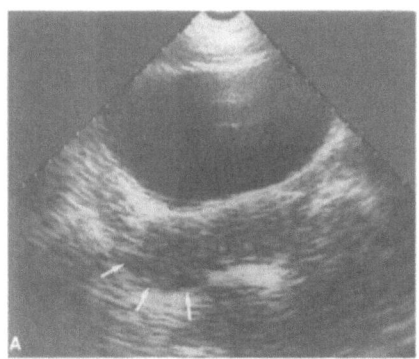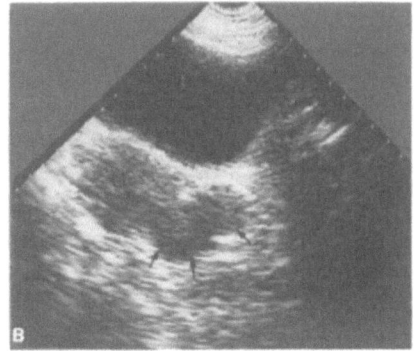

FIG. 21.2.2. ENDOMETRIOSIS

(A,B) Transverse sector scans visualizing adenexal masses (arrows), which are difficult to separate from normal pelvic anatomy. Bladder (B), uterus (U).

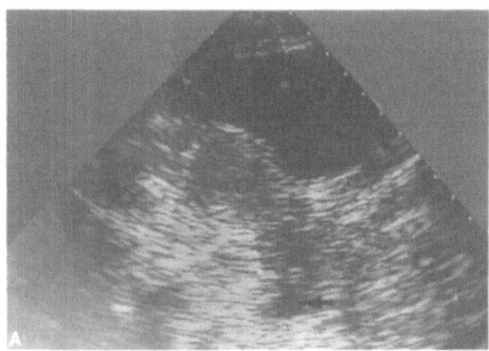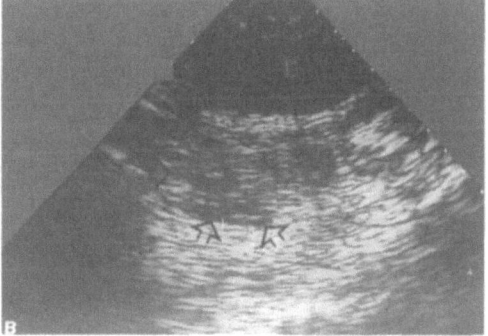

FIG. 21.2.3. PELVIC INFLAMMATORY DISEASE (PID)

(A) Longitudinal scan showing bladder (B), uterus (U), and an irregular mass in the cul de sac (arrow) which has high- and low-level echoes.

(B) Transverse scan of PID (open arrows). Note the difficulty in separating the uterus (U) and adnexal anatomy.

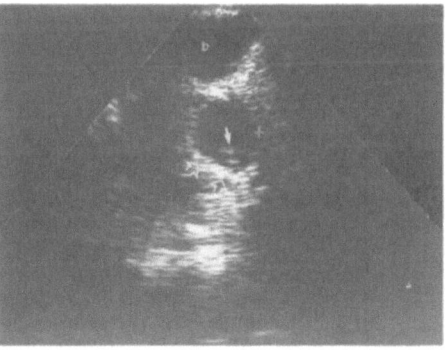

FIG. 21.2.4. TUBO-OVARIAN ABSCESS (TOA)

Longitudinal scan showing a TOA. Note the thickened border (open arrow) with internal echoes (arrow) showing fluid level. Bladder (b).

CHAPTER 21 • ABNORMAL PELVIC ANATOMY

21.2.2. Ovarian Pathology

- Sonography is not meant to replace histopathology in the differential diagnosis of an adnexal mass. Rather, sonography is to be used within its capabilities to identify the presence of an abnormal mass and define the size, shape, location, and internal acoustic characteristics.

- While these parameters may at times permit establishment of a differential diagnosis, it must be recognized that the purpose of sonography is not to establish, but to aid in making, a differential diagnosis.

- The function of sonography is thus *descriptive* and not *diagnostic* in most instances.

- A major consideration is the sonographic determination of ovarian masses. While a definite diagnosis cannot be made sonographically, certain rules of differentiation apply:

    o The more bizarre the sonographic appearance of the mass, the more likely the potential for malignancy (refer to Fig. 21.2.10).
    o If mobile more likely benign, if fixed more likely malignant.
    o The more ascites (see Chapter 22), the more likely a malignancy.
    o The less distinct the outer limits of a mass, the larger the likelihood of malignancy.

- Ovarian masses may have any of several forms:

Cystic (fluid filled):

    o Sonographically characterized by a clear outline, smooth thin walls, anechoic texture, and *good* transonicity (see Fig. 21.2.5).
    o If only a single cystic structure is seen, include follicular cysts, corpus luteum cysts, fimbrial and paraovarian cysts, and serous cystadenoma. When multiple cystic structures are seen (*septae*) the differential diagnosis may include endometriomas (Section 21.2.1), theca-lutein cysts, dermoid cysts, (Chapter 15), polycystic ovaries, and mucinous cystadenoma (see Fig. 21.2.6).

Solid:

    o Sonographically characterized by poorly defined to nonexistent posterior borders, finely or coarsely echo filled, and *poor* transonicity. Acoustic shadowing will increase as density of the mass increases (see Fig. 21.2.8).
    o These include fibromas (see Fig. 21.2.7.), thecomas, Brenner tumors, metastatic lesions (giving a bull's eye appearance), hilar cell tumors, dysgerminomas, and other solid malignant tumors of the ovary.

Complex (combination of cystic and solid components) (see Fig. 21.2.7):

    o The complex appearance of these masses results from echogenicity of septae, blood, puss, mucin, dermoid elements, and other components.
    o These masses may represent benign and malignant cystic teratomas (see Figs. 21.2.8 and 21.2.9), various ovarian carcinomas, granulosa-theca cell tumors, gonadoblastomas and other germ cell tumors, and Kruckenberg tumors (usually bilateral).

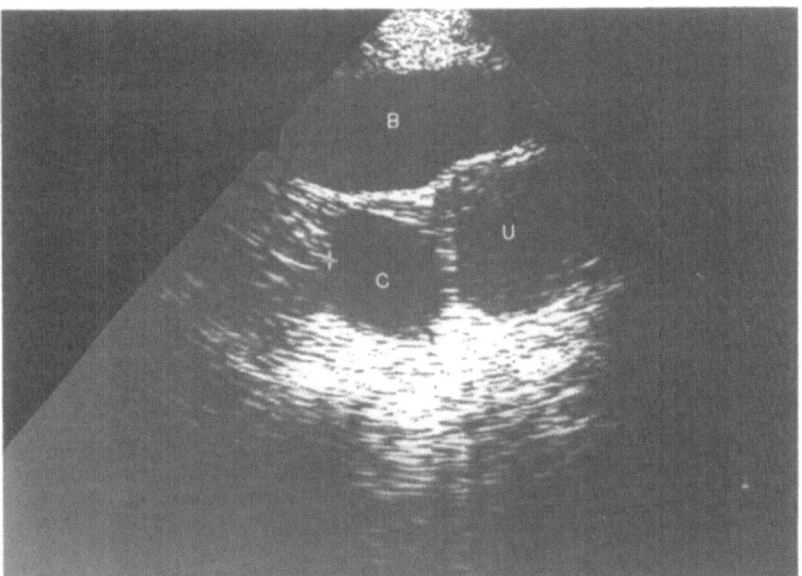

FIG. 21.2.5. SIMPLE OVARIAN CYST

Transverse sector scan demonstrating an ovarian cyst (C). Note the anechoic appearance, smooth borders, and increased transonicity typical of a simple cyst. Bladder (B), uterus (U).

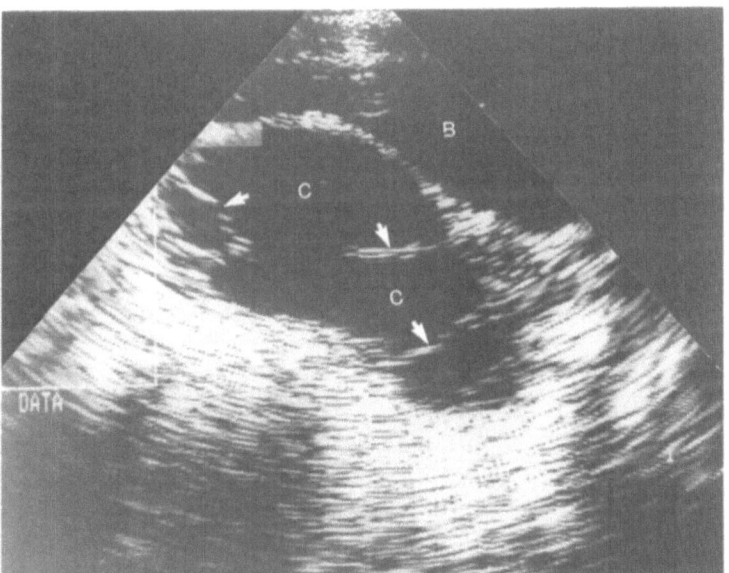

FIG. 21.2.6. SEROUS CYSTADENOMA

Longitudinal sector scan demonstrating a multiloculated cyst showing multiple septae (arrows). The pathology report for this patient was serous cystadenoma. Note the characteristic increase in transonicity. Bladder (B), cystic components (C).

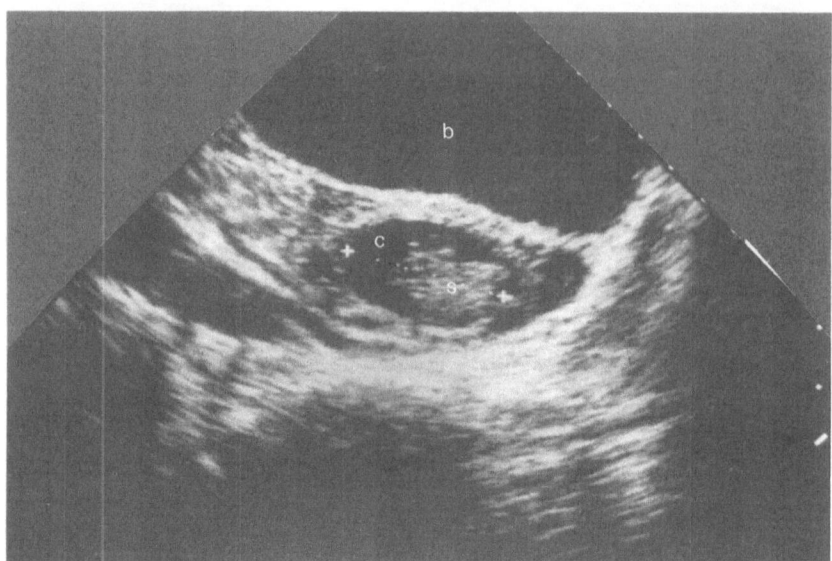

FIG. 21.2.7. COMPLEX OVARIAN TUMOR

Longitudinal sector scan of an ovarian mass (calipers) demonstrating cystic (c) as well as solid (s) areas. Bladder (b).

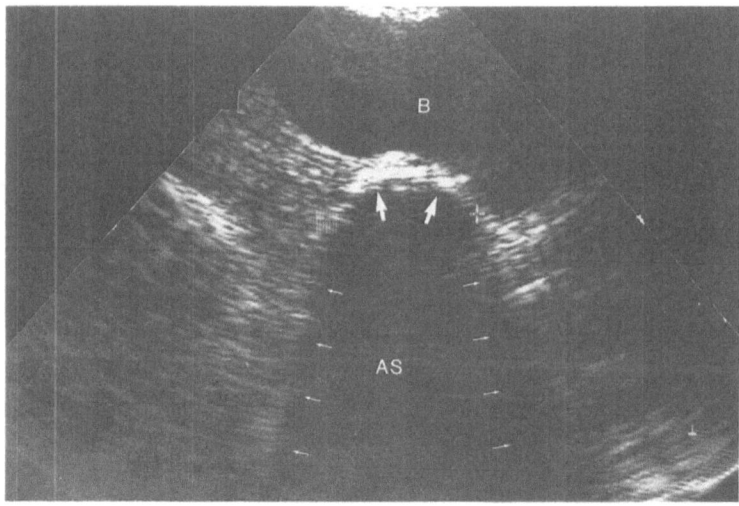

FIG. 21.2.8. SOLID OVARIAN TUMOR

Longitudinal sector scan demonstrating acoustic shadowing (AS, small arrows) from a solid ovarian tumor. Note that no posterior border is visualized. The bright echo (large arrows) represents the beginning of the mass. Bladder (B).

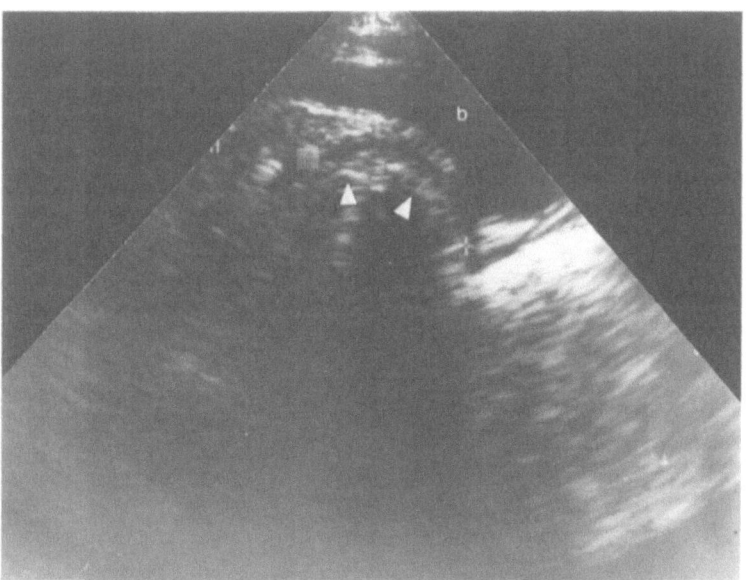

FIG. 21.2.9. BENIGN CYSTIC TERATOMA (BCT)

Longitudinal scan depicting a BCT. Calipers indicate the size of the mass while the arrowheads point to the characteristic "tip of the iceberg" appearance due to dermoid elements. Bladder (b).

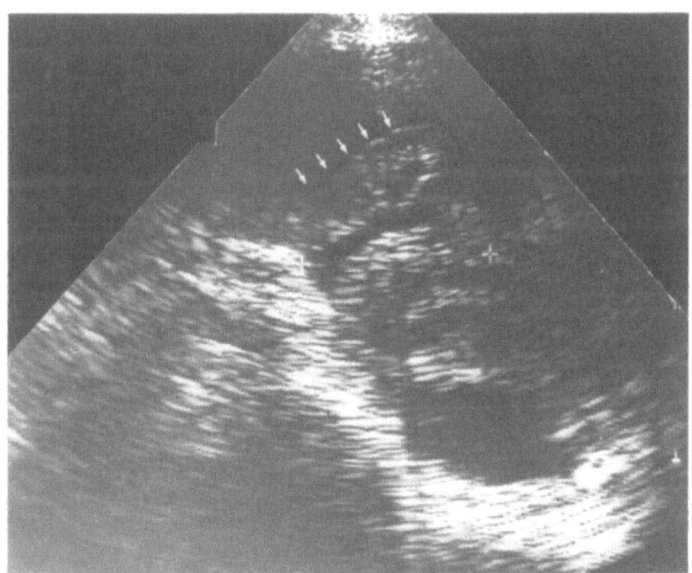

FIG. 21.2.10. OVARIAN CARCINOMA

Longitudinal scan of an ovarian mass, which fills the entire scan. Note the bizarre appearance (complex) and projections (arrows) into the mass.

Chapter 22
Nongynecologic Pelvic Sonography

- Real-time sonography of the pelvis includes the recognition and evauation of nongynecologic structures.

- For example, identification of bowel loops has become extremely simple through direct visualization of *peristalsis* with real-time equipment (see Fig. 22.1.1).

- Other structures and/or pathologic entities that may have to be evaluated via pelvic ultrasound include the following:

  o Pelvic kidney
     Sonographic appearance is that of a normal kidney with calyces pointing posteriorly. (See Fig. 22.1.2.)
  o Mesenteric cysts
  o Appendicular abscesses
  o Diverticular abscesses
  o Abdominal wall hematomas
  o Hematomas
     Many arise from various organs. Sonographic appearance will vary from cystic (in early stages) to a more homogeneous appearance with increasing organization.

- Gynecologic urologic evaluation are presently in an investigative stage.

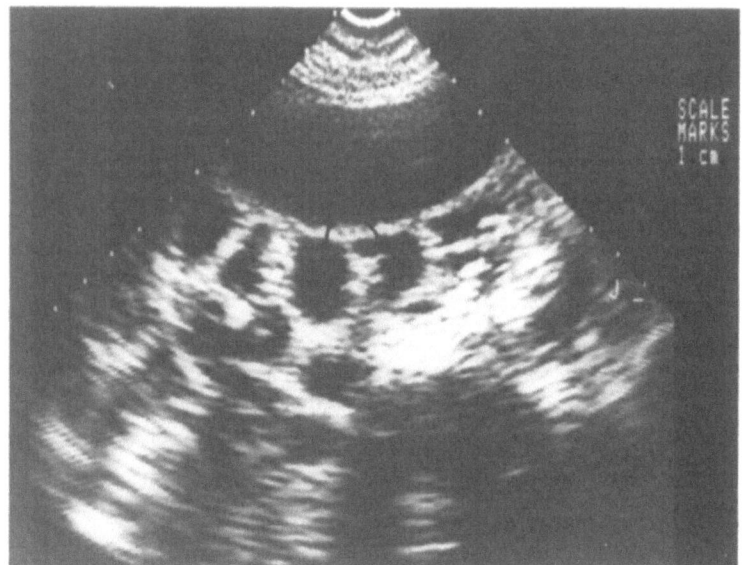

FIG. 22.1.1. NORMAL BOWEL LOOPS IN PELVIS

Transverse scan of the pelvis. Arrows point to loops of bowel that can be misdiagnosed as a multiloculated cyst. Real-time sonography affords quick differentiation due to peristalsis within these areas. Bladder (B).

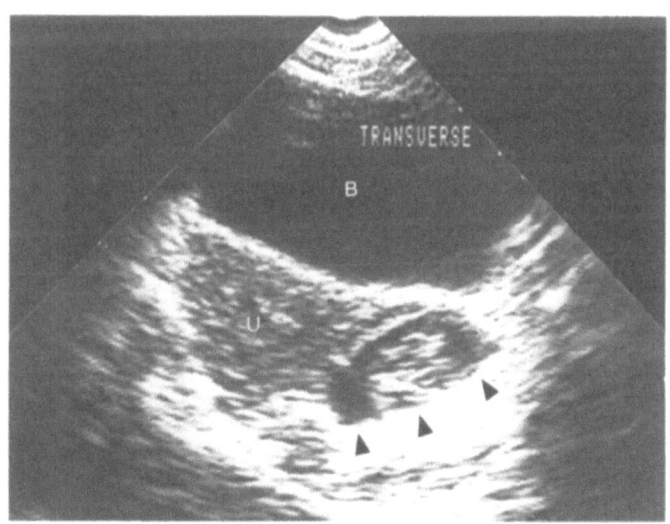

FIG. 22.1.2. PELVIC KIDNEY

Transverse scan of pelvic kidney (arrowheads). Note the posterior position of the pelvio-caliceal echoes. Uterus (U), bladder (B).

CHAPTER 22 • NONGYNECOLOGIC PELVIC SONOGRAPHY   **215**

Chapter 23
Ascites

- A small amount of peritoneal fluid in the cul de sac is normal.

- This amount may be increased with acute intraabdominal processes such as pelvic inflammatory disease (PID). At what point the term "ascites" should be used rather than the term "excessive peritoneal fluid" has not been defined.

- Ascites also needs to be differentiated from a hemoperitoneum, which may be impossible in the early stages of a hemoperitoneum.

- Once ascites is diagnosed, the main sonographic concern is the differentiation of *benign* (see Fig. 23.1.1.) from *malignant* ascites.

- The main characteristics differentiating benign from malignant ascites are listed in Table 23.1.1.[1]

TABLE 23.1.1.

Characteristics of Benign and Malignant Ascites[a]

Benign	Malignant
Large sonolucent areas without apparent borders	Bizarre sonographic pattern (echogenic opacities mixed with sonolucent areas)
Usually in lower areas of peritoneal cavity with free-floating bowel (see Fig. 23.1.1)	Intestines fixed dorsally, with fluid pockets anteriorly
Change of fluid levels with tiltings of the patient (see Fig. 23.1.2)	Fluid levels fixed with tilting of the patient

[a]Modified from Sanders and James.[1]

REFERENCES

1. Sanders RC, James AE: *Ultrasonography in Obstetrics and Gynecology.* East Norwalk, Connecticut, Appleton-Century-Crofts, 1977, p. 307.

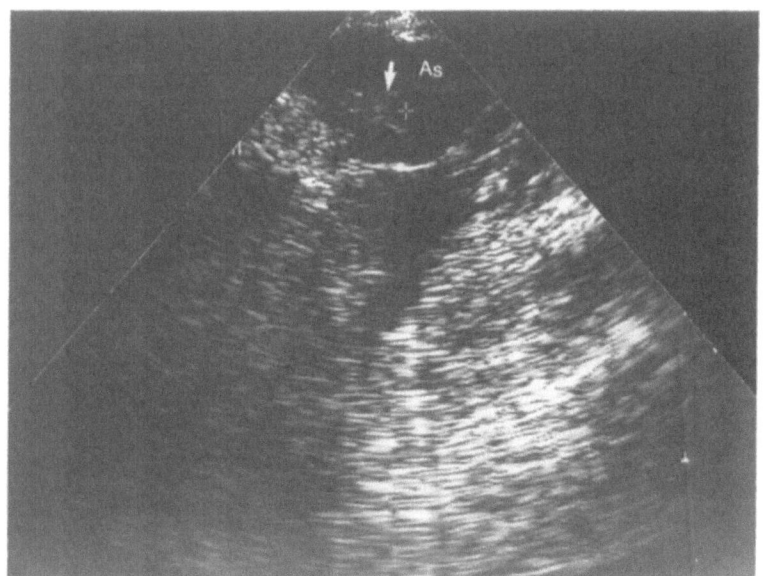

FIG. 23.1.1. BENIGN ASCITES

Transverse sector scan demonstrating free-floating bowel loops (arrow) in benign ascites (As).

Index

Index

TABLE 8.2.1

Estimated Fetal Weights[a]

Biparietal diameters	Abdominal circumferences																																																	
	15.5	16.0	16.5	17.0	17.5	18.0	18.5	19.0	19.5	20.0	20.5	21.0	21.5	22.0	22.5	23.0	23.5	24.0	24.5	25.0	25.5	26.0	26.5	27.0	27.5	28.0	28.5	29.0	29.5	30.0	30.5	31.0	31.5	32.0	32.5	33.0	33.5	34.0	34.5	35.0	35.5	36.0	36.5	37.0	37.5	38.0	38.5	39.0	39.5	40.0
3.1	224	234	244	255	267	279	291	304	318	332	346	362	378	395	412	431	450	470	491	513	536	559	584	610	638	666	696	726	759	793	828	865	903	943	985	1,029	1,075	1,123	1,173	1,225	1,279	1,336	1,396	1,458	1,523	1,591	1,661	1,735	1,812	1,893
3.2	231	241	251	263	274	286	299	312	326	340	355	371	388	405	423	441	461	481	502	525	548	572	597	624	651	680	710	742	774	809	844	882	921	961	1,004	1,048	1,094	1,143	1,193	1,246	1,301	1,358	1,418	1,481	1,546	1,615	1,686	1,761	1,838	1,920
3.3	237	248	259	270	282	294	307	321	335	349	365	381	397	415	433	452	472	493	514	537	560	585	611	638	666	695	725	757	790	825	861	899	938	979	1,022	1,067	1,114	1,163	1,214	1,267	1,323	1,381	1,441	1,504	1,570	1,639	1,711	1,786	1,865	1,946
3.4	244	255	266	278	290	302	316	329	344	359	374	391	408	425	444	463	483	504	526	549	573	598	624	652	680	710	740	773	806	841	878	916	956	998	1,041	1,087	1,134	1,183	1,235	1,289	1,345	1,403	1,464	1,528	1,595	1,664	1,737	1,812	1,891	1,973
3.5	251	262	274	285	298	311	324	338	353	368	384	401	418	436	455	475	495	517	539	562	587	612	638	666	695	725	756	789	823	858	896	934	975	1,017	1,061	1,107	1,154	1,204	1,256	1,311	1,367	1,426	1,488	1,552	1,619	1,689	1,762	1,839	1,918	2,001
3.6	259	270	281	294	306	319	333	347	362	378	394	411	429	447	466	486	507	529	552	575	600	626	653	681	710	740	772	805	840	876	913	953	993	1,036	1,080	1,127	1,175	1,226	1,278	1,333	1,390	1,450	1,512	1,577	1,645	1,715	1,789	1,865	1,945	2,029
3.7	266	278	290	302	315	328	342	357	372	388	404	422	440	458	478	498	519	542	565	589	614	640	667	696	725	756	788	822	857	893	931	971	1,012	1,056	1,101	1,147	1,196	1,247	1,300	1,356	1,413	1,474	1,536	1,602	1,670	1,741	1,815	1,893	1,973	2,057
3.8	274	286	298	310	324	337	352	366	382	398	415	432	451	470	490	510	532	554	578	602	628	654	682	711	741	772	805	839	874	911	950	990	1,032	1,076	1,121	1,168	1,218	1,269	1,323	1,379	1,437	1,498	1,561	1,627	1,696	1,768	1,842	1,920	2,001	2,086
3.9	282	294	306	319	333	347	361	376	392	409	426	444	462	482	502	523	545	568	592	616	642	669	697	727	757	789	822	856	892	930	969	1,009	1,052	1,096	1,142	1,190	1,240	1,292	1,346	1,402	1,461	1,523	1,586	1,653	1,722	1,794	1,870	1,948	2,030	2,115
4.0	290	303	315	328	342	356	371	386	403	419	437	455	474	494	514	536	558	581	606	631	657	684	713	743	773	806	839	874	911	949	988	1,029	1,072	1,117	1,163	1,212	1,262	1,315	1,369	1,426	1,486	1,548	1,612	1,679	1,749	1,822	1,898	1,977	2,059	2,145
4.1	299	311	324	338	352	366	381	397	413	430	448	467	486	506	527	549	572	595	620	645	672	700	729	759	790	828	857	892	929	968	1,008	1,049	1,093	1,138	1,185	1,234	1,285	1,338	1,393	1,451	1,511	1,573	1,638	1,706	1,776	1,849	1,926	2,005	2,088	2,174
4.2	308	320	333	347	361	376	392	408	424	442	460	479	498	519	540	562	585	609	634	660	688	716	745	776	807	841	875	911	948	987	1,028	1,070	1,114	1,159	1,207	1,256	1,308	1,361	1,417	1,475	1,536	1,599	1,664	1,733	1,804	1,878	1,954	2,035	2,118	2,205
4.3	317	330	343	357	371	387	402	419	436	453	472	491	511	532	554	576	600	624	649	676	703	732	762	793	825	859	893	930	968	1,007	1,048	1,091	1,135	1,181	1,229	1,279	1,331	1,385	1,442	1,500	1,562	1,625	1,691	1,760	1,832	1,906	1,984	2,064	2,148	2,236
4.4	326	339	353	367	382	397	413	430	447	465	484	504	524	545	567	590	614	639	665	692	719	749	779	810	843	877	912	949	987	1,027	1,069	1,112	1,157	1,204	1,252	1,303	1,355	1,410	1,467	1,526	1,588	1,652	1,718	1,788	1,860	1,935	2,013	2,094	2,179	2,267
4.5	335	349	363	377	393	408	425	442	459	478	497	517	538	559	581	605	629	654	680	708	736	765	796	828	861	896	932	969	1,008	1,048	1,090	1,134	1,179	1,226	1,275	1,326	1,380	1,435	1,492	1,552	1,614	1,679	1,746	1,816	1,889	1,964	2,043	2,125	2,210	2,298
4.6	345	359	373	388	404	420	436	454	472	490	510	530	551	573	596	620	644	670	696	724	753	783	814	846	880	915	951	989	1,028	1,069	1,112	1,156	1,202	1,249	1,299	1,351	1,404	1,460	1,518	1,579	1,641	1,706	1,774	1,845	1,918	1,994	2,073	2,156	2,241	2,330
4.7	355	369	384	399	415	431	448	466	484	503	523	544	565	588	611	635	660	686	713	741	770	801	832	865	899	934	971	1,010	1,049	1,091	1,134	1,178	1,225	1,273	1,323	1,375	1,430	1,486	1,545	1,605	1,669	1,734	1,803	1,874	1,948	2,024	2,104	2,187	2,273	2,363
4.8	366	380	395	410	426	443	460	478	497	517	537	558	580	602	626	650	676	702	730	758	788	819	851	884	919	954	992	1,031	1,071	1,113	1,156	1,201	1,248	1,297	1,348	1,401	1,455	1,512	1,571	1,633	1,697	1,763	1,832	1,904	1,978	2,055	2,136	2,219	2,306	2,396
4.9	379	391	406	422	438	455	473	491	510	530	551	572	594	617	641	666	692	719	747	776	806	837	870	903	938	975	1,013	1,052	1,093	1,135	1,179	1,225	1,272	1,322	1,373	1,426	1,482	1,539	1,599	1,661	1,725	1,792	1,861	1,934	2,009	2,086	2,167	2,251	2,339	2,429
5.0	387	402	418	434	451	468	486	505	524	544	565	587	610	633	657	683	709	736	765	794	824	856	889	923	959	996	1,034	1,074	1,115	1,158	1,203	1,249	1,297	1,347	1,399	1,452	1,508	1,566	1,626	1,689	1,754	1,821	1,891	1,964	2,040	2,118	2,200	2,284	2,372	2,463
5.1	399	414	430	446	463	481	499	518	538	559	580	602	625	649	674	699	726	754	783	812	843	876	909	944	980	1,017	1,056	1,096	1,138	1,181	1,226	1,273	1,322	1,372	1,425	1,479	1,535	1,594	1,655	1,718	1,783	1,851	1,922	1,995	2,071	2,150	2,232	2,317	2,406	2,498
5.2	410	426	442	459	476	494	513	532	552	573	595	618	641	665	690	717	744	772	801	831	863	895	929	964	1,001	1,039	1,078	1,119	1,161	1,205	1,251	1,298	1,347	1,398	1,451	1,506	1,563	1,622	1,683	1,747	1,813	1,882	1,953	2,027	2,103	2,183	2,266	2,351	2,440	2,532
5.3	422	438	455	472	489	508	527	547	567	589	611	634	657	682	708	734	762	790	820	851	883	916	950	986	1,023	1,061	1,101	1,142	1,185	1,229	1,276	1,323	1,373	1,425	1,478	1,533	1,591	1,651	1,713	1,777	1,843	1,913	1,984	2,059	2,136	2,216	2,299	2,386	2,475	2,568
5.4	435	451	468	485	503	522	541	561	582	604	627	650	674	699	725	752	780	809	839	870	903	936	971	1,007	1,045	1,084	1,124	1,166	1,209	1,254	1,301	1,349	1,399	1,452	1,506	1,562	1,620	1,680	1,742	1,807	1,874	1,944	2,016	2,091	2,169	2,250	2,333	2,420	2,510	2,604
5.5	447	464	481	499	517	536	556	577	598	620	643	667	691	717	743	771	799	828	859	891	924	958	993	1,030	1,068	1,107	1,148	1,190	1,234	1,279	1,327	1,376	1,426	1,479	1,534	1,590	1,649	1,710	1,773	1,838	1,906	1,976	2,049	2,124	2,203	2,284	2,368	2,456	2,546	2,640
5.6	461	477	495	513	532	551	571	592	614	636	660	684	709	735	762	789	818	848	879	911	945	979	1,015	1,052	1,091	1,131	1,172	1,215	1,259	1,305	1,353	1,402	1,454	1,507	1,562	1,619	1,678	1,740	1,803	1,869	1,938	2,008	2,082	2,158	2,237	2,319	2,403	2,491	2,582	2,677
5.7	474	491	509	527	547	566	587	608	630	653	677	701	727	753	780	809	838	869	900	933	966	1,001	1,038	1,075	1,114	1,155	1,197	1,240	1,285	1,332	1,380	1,430	1,482	1,535	1,591	1,649	1,709	1,770	1,835	1,901	1,970	2,041	2,115	2,192	2,272	2,354	2,439	2,528	2,619	2,714
5.8	488	505	524	542	562	582	603	625	647	670	695	719	745	772	800	829	858	889	921	954	989	1,024	1,061	1,099	1,139	1,180	1,222	1,266	1,311	1,358	1,407	1,458	1,510	1,564	1,621	1,679	1,739	1,802	1,866	1,934	2,003	2,075	2,150	2,227	2,307	2,390	2,475	2,564	2,657	2,752
5.9	502	520	539	558	578	598	619	642	664	688	713	738	764	792	820	849	879	911	943	977	1,011	1,047	1,085	1,123	1,163	1,205	1,248	1,292	1,338	1,386	1,435	1,486	1,539	1,594	1,651	1,710	1,770	1,834	1,899	1,966	2,037	2,109	2,184	2,262	2,342	2,426	2,512	2,602	2,694	2,790
6.0	517	535	554	573	594	615	636	659	682	706	731	757	784	811	840	870	900	932	965	999	1,035	1,071	1,109	1,148	1,189	1,231	1,274	1,319	1,366	1,414	1,464	1,515	1,569	1,624	1,682	1,741	1,802	1,866	1,932	2,000	2,071	2,144	2,219	2,298	2,379	2,463	2,550	2,640	2,733	2,829
6.1	532	550	570	590	610	632	654	677	700	725	750	777	804	832	861	891	922	955	988	1,023	1,058	1,095	1,134	1,173	1,214	1,257	1,301	1,346	1,393	1,442	1,493	1,545	1,599	1,655	1,713	1,773	1,835	1,899	1,965	2,034	2,105	2,179	2,255	2,334	2,416	2,500	2,588	2,678	2,772	2,869
6.2	547	566	586	606	627	649	672	695	719	744	770	797	824	853	882	913	945	977	1,011	1,046	1,083	1,120	1,159	1,199	1,241	1,284	1,328	1,374	1,422	1,471	1,522	1,575	1,630	1,686	1,745	1,805	1,868	1,932	1,999	2,069	2,140	2,215	2,291	2,371	2,453	2,538	2,626	2,717	2,811	2,909
6.3	563	583	603	624	645	667	690	714	738	764	790	817	845	874	904	935	967	1,001	1,035	1,071	1,107	1,145	1,185	1,226	1,268	1,311	1,356	1,403	1,451	1,501	1,552	1,606	1,661	1,718	1,777	1,838	1,901	1,967	2,034	2,104	2,176	2,251	2,328	2,408	2,491	2,577	2,665	2,757	2,851	2,949
6.4	580	600	620	641	663	686	709	733	758	784	811	838	867	896	927	958	991	1,025	1,059	1,096	1,133	1,171	1,211	1,253	1,295	1,339	1,385	1,432	1,481	1,531	1,583	1,637	1,693	1,751	1,810	1,872	1,935	2,001	2,069	2,140	2,213	2,288	2,366	2,446	2,530	2,616	2,705	2,797	2,892	2,991
6.5	597	617	638	659	682	705	728	753	778	805	832	860	889	919	950	982	1,015	1,049	1,084	1,121	1,159	1,198	1,238	1,280	1,323	1,368	1,414	1,462	1,511	1,562	1,615	1,669	1,725	1,784	1,844	1,906	1,970	2,037	2,105	2,176	2,250	2,326	2,404	2,485	2,569	2,656	2,745	2,838	2,933	3,032
6.6	614	635	656	678	701	724	748	773	799	826	853	882	911	942	973	1,006	1,039	1,074	1,110	1,147	1,185	1,225	1,266	1,308	1,352	1,397	1,444	1,492	1,542	1,594	1,647	1,702	1,759	1,817	1,878	1,941	2,006	2,073	2,142	2,213	2,287	2,364	2,443	2,524	2,609	2,696	2,786	2,879	2,975	3,075
6.7	632	653	675	697	720	744	769	794	820	848	876	905	935	965	997	1,030	1,065	1,100	1,136	1,174	1,213	1,253	1,294	1,337	1,381	1,427	1,474	1,523	1,574	1,626	1,679	1,735	1,792	1,852	1,913	1,976	2,042	2,109	2,179	2,251	2,326	2,403	2,482	2,564	2,649	2,737	2,827	2,921	3,018	3,117
6.8	651	672	694	717	740	765	790	816	842	870	898	928	958	990	1,022	1,056	1,090	1,126	1,163	1,201	1,241	1,281	1,323	1,367	1,411	1,458	1,505	1,555	1,606	1,658	1,713	1,769	1,827	1,887	1,949	2,012	2,078	2,147	2,217	2,290	2,365	2,442	2,522	2,605	2,690	2,778	2,869	2,964	3,061	3,161
6.9	670	691	714	737	761	786	811	838	865	893	922	952	983	1,015	1,048	1,082	1,117	1,153	1,190	1,229	1,269	1,310	1,353	1,397	1,442	1,489	1,537	1,587	1,639	1,692	1,747	1,803	1,862	1,922	1,985	2,049	2,116	2,184	2,255	2,329	2,404	2,482	2,563	2,646	2,732	2,821	2,912	3,007	3,104	3,205
7.0	689	711	734	758	782	807	833	860	888	916	946	976	1,008	1,040	1,074	1,108	1,144	1,181	1,219	1,258	1,298	1,340	1,383	1,427	1,473	1,521	1,570	1,620	1,672	1,726	1,781	1,839	1,898	1,959	2,022	2,087	2,154	2,223	2,295	2,368	2,444	2,523	2,604	2,688	2,774	2,863	2,955	3,050	3,149	3,250
7.1	709	732	755	779	804	830	856	883	912	941	971	1,002	1,033	1,066	1,100	1,135	1,171	1,209	1,247	1,287	1,328	1,370	1,414	1,459	1,505	1,553	1,603	1,654	1,706	1,761	1,817	1,875	1,934	1,996	2,059	2,125	2,193	2,262	2,334	2,409	2,485	2,564	2,646	2,730	2,817	2,907	2,999	3,095	3,193	3,295
7.2	730	763	777	801	827	853	880	907	936	965	996	1,027	1,060	1,093	1,128	1,163	1,200	1,238	1,277	1,317	1,358	1,401	1,445	1,491	1,538	1,586	1,636	1,688	1,741	1,796	1,853	1,911	1,971	2,044	2,098	2,164	2,232	2,302	2,375	2,450	2,527	2,607	2,689	2,773	2,861	2,951	3,044	3,140	3,239	3,341
7.3	751	775	799	824	850	876	904	932	961	991	1,022	1,054	1,087	1,121	1,156	1,192	1,229	1,267	1,307	1,348	1,390	1,433	1,478	1,524	1,571	1,620	1,671	1,723	1,777	1,832	1,890	1,948	2,009	2,072	2,137	2,203	2,272	2,343	2,416	2,491	2,569	2,649	2,732	2,817	2,905	2,996	3,089	3,186	3,285	3,388
7.4	773	797	822	847	874	901	928	957	987	1,017	1,049	1,081	1,114	1,149	1,184	1,221	1,259	1,297	1,338	1,379	1,421	1,465	1,511	1,557	1,605	1,655	1,706	1,759	1,813	1,869	1,927	1,987	2,048	2,111	2,176	2,244	2,313	2,384	2,458	2,534	2,612	2,693	2,776	2,862	2,950	3,041	3,135	3,232	3,332	3,435
7.5	796	820	845	871	898	925	954	983	1,013	1,044	1,076	1,109	1,143	1,178	1,214	1,251	1,289	1,328	1,369	1,411	1,454	1,499	1,544	1,592	1,640	1,690	1,742	1,795	1,850	1,907	1,965	2,025	2,087	2,151	2,217	2,265	2,354	2,426	2,501	2,577	2,656	2,737	2,821	2,907	2,996	3,088	3,182	3,279	3,380	3,483
7.6	819	844	870	896	923	951	980	1,009	1,040	1,072	1,104	1,137	1,172	1,207	1,244	1,281	1,320	1,360	1,401	1,444	1,487	1,533	1,579	1,627	1,676	1,727	1,779	1,833	1,888	1,945	2,004	2,065	2,127	2,192	2,258	2,326	2,397	2,469	2,544	2,621	2,700	2,782	2,866	2,953	3,042	3,134	3,229	3,327	3,428	3,531
7.7	843	868	894	921	949	977	1,007	1,037	1,068	1,100	1,133	1,167	1,202	1,238	1,275	1,313	1,352	1,393	1,434	1,477	1,522	1,567	1,614	1,663	1,712	1,764	1,816	1,871	1,927	1,985	2,044	2,105	2,168	2,233	2,300	2,369	2,440	2,513	2,588	2,666	2,746	2,828	2,912	3,000	3,090	3,182	3,277	3,376	3,477	3,581
7.8	868	894	920	947	975	1,004	1,034	1,065	1,096	1,129	1,162	1,197	1,232	1,269	1,306	1,345	1,385	1,426	1,468	1,512	1,557	1,603	1,650	1,699	1,749	1,801	1,855	1,910	1,966	2,025	2,085	2,146	2,210	2,275	2,343	2,412	2,484	2,557	2,633	2,711	2,792	2,874	2,959	3,047	3,137	3,230	3,326	3,425	3,526	3,631
7.9	893	919	946	974	1,003	1,032	1,062	1,094	1,126	1,159	1,193	1,228	1,264	1,301	1,339	1,378	1,418	1,460	1,503	1,547	1,592	1,639	1,687	1,737	1,787	1,840	1,894	1,949	2,006	2,065	2,126	2,188	2,252	2,318	2,386	2,456	2,528	2,603	2,679	2,757	2,838	2,921	3,007	3,095	3,186	3,279	3,376	3,475	3,576	3,681
8.0	919	946	973	1,002	1,031	1,061	1,091	1,123	1,156	1,189	1,224	1,259	1,296	1,333	1,372	1,412	1,453	1,495	1,538	1,583	1,629	1,676	1,725	1,775	1,826	1,879	1,934	1,990	2,048	2,107	2,168	2,231	2,296	2,362	2,431	2,501	2,574	2,649	2,725	2,804	2,886	2,969	3,056	3,144	3,235	3,329	3,426	3,525	3,627	3,733
8.1	946	973	1,001	1,030	1,060	1,090	1,121	1,153	1,187	1,221	1,256	1,292	1,329	1,367	1,406	1,446	1,488	1,531	1,575	1,620	1,666	1,714	1,763	1,814	1,866	1,919	1,975	2,031	2,089	2,149	2,211	2,275	2,340	2,407	2,476	2,547	2,620	2,695	2,773	2,852	2,934	3,018	3,105	3,194	3,286	3,380	3,477	3,577	3,679	3,785
8.2	974	1,001	1,030	1,059	1,089	1,120	1,152	1,185	1,218	1,253	1,288	1,325	1,363	1,401	1,441	1,482	1,524	1,567	1,612	1,657	1,704	1,753	1,803	1,854	1,906	1,960	2,016	2,073	2,132	2,193	2,255	2,319	2,385	2,462	2,522	2,594	2,667	2,743	2,821	2,901	2,983	3,068	3,155	3,244	3,336	3,431	3,529	3,629	3,732	3,838
8.3	1,002	1,030	1,059	1,089	1,120	1,151	1,183	1,217	1,251	1,286	1,322	1,359	1,397	1,436	1,477	1,518	1,561	1,605	1,650	1,696	1,744	1,793	1,843	1,895	1,948	2,002	2,059	2,116	2,176	2,237	2,300	2,364	2,431	2,499	2,569	2,641	2,715	2,791	2,870	2,950	3,033	3,118	3,206	3,296	3,388	3,483	3,581	3,682	3,785	3,891
8.4	1,032	1,060	1,090	1,120	1,151	1,183	1,216	1,249	1,284	1,320	1,356	1,394	1,433	1,473	1,513	1,555	1,599	1,643	1,689	1,735	1,784	1,833	1,884	1,936	1,990	2,045	2,102	2,160	2,220	2,282	2,345	2,410	2,477	2,546	2,617	2,689	2,764	2,841	2,920	3,001	3,084	3,169	3,257	3,348	3,441	3,536	3,634	3,735	3,839	3,945
8.5	1,062	1,091	1,121	1,151	1,183	1,216	1,249	1,283	1,318	1,355	1,392	1,430	1,469	1,510	1,551	1,594	1,637	1,682	1,728	1,776	1,825	1,875	1,926	1,979	2,033	2,089	2,146	2,205	2,266	2,328	2,392	2,457	2,525	2,594	2,665	2,739	2,814	2,891	2,970	3,052	3,135	3,221	3,310	3,401	3,494	3,590	3,688	3,790	3,894	4,000
8.6	1,093	1,122	1,153	1,184	1,216	1,249	1,283	1,318	1,354	1,390	1,428	1,467	1,507	1,548	1,589	1,633	1,677	1,722	1,769	1,817	1,866	1,917	1,969	2,022	2,077	2,134	2,192	2,251	2,312	2,375	2,439	2,505	2,573	2,643	2,715	2,789	2,864	2,942	3,022	3,104	3,188	3,274	3,363	3,454	3,548	3,644	3,743	3,845	3,949	4,056
8.7	1,125	1,155	1,186	1,218	1,250	1,284	1,318	1,353	1,390	1,427	1,465	1,505	1,545	1,586	1,629	1,673	1,717	1,764	1,811	1,859	1,909	1,960	2,013	2,067	2,122	2,179	2,238	2,298	2,359	2,423	2,488	2,554	2,623	2,693	2,765	2,840	2,916	2,994	3,074	3,157	3,241	3,328	3,417	3,509	3,603	3,700	3,799	3,901	4,005	4,113
8.8	1,157	1,188	1,220	1,252	1,285	1,319	1,354	1,390	1,427	1,465	1,504	1,543	1,584	1,626	1,669	1,714	1,759	1,806	1,854	1,903	1,953	2,005	2,058	2,113	2,169	2,226	2,285	2,346	2,408	2,472	2,537	2,604	2,673	2,744	2,817	2,892	2,968	3,047	3,128	3,210	3,295	3,383	3,472	3,565	3,659	3,756	3,855	3,958	4,063	4,170
8.9	1,191	1,222	1,254	1,287	1,321	1,356	1,391	1,428	1,465	1,503	1,543	1,583	1,625	1,667	1,711	1,756	1,802	1,849	1,897	1,947	1,998	2,050	2,104	2,159	2,216	2,274	2,333	2,394	2,457	2,521	2,587	2,655	2,725	2,796	2,869	2,944	3,021	3,101	3,182	3,265	3,351	3,438	3,528	3,621	3,716	3,813	3,913	4,015	4,120	4,228
9.0	1,226	1,258	1,290	1,324	1,358	1,393	1,429	1,456	1,504	1,543	1,583	1,624	1,666	1,709	1,753	1,799	1,845	1,893	1,942	1,992	2,044	2,097	2,151	2,207	2,264	2,322	2,382	2,444	2,507	2,572	2,639	2,707	2,777	2,849	2,923	2,998	3,076	3,155	3,237	3,321	3,407	3,495	3,585	3,678	3,773	3,871	3,971	4,074	4,179	4,287
9.1	1,262	1,294	1,327	1,361	1,396	1,432	1,468	1,506	1,544	1,584	1,624	1,666	1,708	1,752	1,797	1,843	1,890	1,938	1,988	2,039	2,091	2,144	2,199	2,255	2,313	2,372	2,433	2,495	2,559	2,624	2,691	2,760	2,830	2,903	2,977	3,053	3,131	3,211	3,293	3,377	3,464	3,552	3,643	3,736	3,832	3,930	4,030	4,133	4,239	4,347
9.2	1,299	1,332	1,365	1,400	1,435	1,471	1,508	1,546	1,586	1,626	1,667	1,709	1,752	1,796	1,841	1,888	1,936	1,984	2,035	2,086	2,139	2,193	2,248	2,305	2,363	2,423	2,484	2,547	2,611	2,677	2,744	2,814	2,885	2,958	3,032	3,109	3,187	3,268	3,350	3,435	3,522	3,611	3,702	3,795	3,891	3,989	4,090	4,193	4,299	4,408
9.3	1,337	1,370	1,404	1,439	1,475	1,512	1,550	1,588	1,628	1,668	1,710	1,753	1,796	1,841	1,887	1,934	1,982	2,032	2,083	2,135	2,188	2,242	2,298	2,356	2,414	2,475	2,536	2,599	2,664	2,731	2,799	2,869	2,940	3,014	3,089	3,166	3,245	3,326	3,409	3,494	3,581	3,670	3,761	3,855	3,951	4,050	4,151	4,254	4,361	4,469
9.4	1,376	1,410	1,444	1,480	1,516	1,554	1,592	1,631	1,671	1,712	1,755	1,798	1,842	1,887	1,934	1,982	2,030	2,080	2,132	2,184	2,238	2,293	2,350	2,407	2,467	2,527	2,590	2,653	2,719	2,786	2,854	2,925	2,997	3,070	3,146	3,224	3,303	3,384	3,468	3,553	3,641	3,738	3,822	3,916	4,013	4,111	4,213	4,316	4,423	4,532
9.5	1,416	1,450	1,486	1,522	1,559	1,597	1,635	1,675	1,716	1,758	1,800	1,844	1,889	1,935	1,982	2,030	2,080	2,130	2,182	2,235	2,289	2,345	2,402	2,460	2,520	2,582	2,644	2,709	2,774	2,842	2,911	2,982	3,054	3,129	3,205	3,283	3,362	3,444	3,528	3,614	3,701	3,791	3,884	3,978	4,075	4,174	4,275	4,379	4,486	4,595
9.6	1,457	1,492	1,528	1,565	1,602	1,641	1,680	1,720	1,762	1,804	1,847	1,892	1,937	1,984	2,031	2,080	2,130	2,181	2,233	2,287	2,342	2,398	2,456	2,515	2,575	2,637	2,700	2,765	2,831	2,899	2,969	3,040	3,113	3,188	3,264	3,343	3,423	3,505	3,589	3,675	3,763	3,854	3,946	4,041	4,138	4,237	4,339	4,443	4,550	4,659
9.7	1,500	1,535	1,572	1,609	1,547	1,686	1,726	1,767	1,809	1,852	1,895	1,940	1,986	2,033	2,082	2,131	2,181	2,233	2,286	2,340	2,396	2,452	2,510	2,570	2,631	2,693	2,757	2,822	2,889	2,958	3,028	3,099	3,173	3,248	3,325	3,404	3,484	3,567	3,651	3,738	3,826	3,917	4,010	4,105	4,202	4,302	4,404	4,508	4,615	4,724
9.8	1,544	1,580	1,617	1,654	1,693	1,733	1,773	1,815	1,857	1,900	1,945	1,990	2,037	2,085	2,133	2,183	2,234	2,286	2,340	2,395	2,451	2,508	2,567	2,627	2,688	2,751	2,815	2,881	2,948	3,017	3,088	3,160	3,234	3,309	3,387	3,466	3,547	3,630	3,715	3,802	3,890	3,981	4,074	4,170	4,267	4,367	4,469	4,573	4,680	4,790
9.9	1,589	1,625	1,663	1,701	1,740	1,781	1,822	1,864	1,907	1,951	1,996	2,042	2,086	2,137	2,186	2,237	2,288	2,341	2,395	2,450	2,507	2,565	2,624	2,684	2,746	2,810	2,874	2,941	3,009	3,078	3,149	3,222	3,296	3,372	3,450	3,529	3,611	3,694	3,779	3,866	3,956	4,047	4,140	4,236	4,333	4,433	4,536	4,640	4,747	4,857
10.0	1,635	1,672	1,710	1,749	1,789	1,830	1,871	1,914	1,958	2,002	2,048	2,094	2,142	2,191	2,241	2,292	2,344	2,397	2,452	2,507	2,564	2,623	2,682	2,743	2,806	2,870	2,935	3,002	3,070	3,140	3,211	3,285	3,359	3,436	3,514	3,594	3,676	3,759	3,845	3,932	4,022	4,113	4,207	4,303	4,400	4,501	4,603	4,708	4,815	4,924

[a]Log (birth weight) = $-1.7942 + 0.166\,(BPD) + 0.032\,(AC) - 2.646\,(BPD) \times AC/1000$.

SD = 106.0 g/kg of body weight. From Shepard *et al.*[1]